CONTENTS

INTRODUCTION

When it comes to digestion, the gastrointestinal tract, which is mostly made up of the digestive system, plays a critical function. This system consists of hollow organs connected by a long, twisting tube that runs from the mouth through the stomach and intestines and finally to the anus. In the human body, it is known as the gastrointestinal tract (GI tract).

Together with the nervous and circular systems, bacteria in the GI tract known as gut flora or microbiome, as well as the digestive organs, digest the food and fluids you consume every time you eat and absorb the nutrients your body requires to function properly and healthily.

The GI tract's functions are, in general, transportation, digestion, and absorption of everything one ingests. However, for these to be met, the sections of the GI must perform their individual functions.

The food should have been broken down into smaller bits by the mouth prior to entering through the esophagus as a food bolus at the beginning of the process. As soon as the food bolus enters the stomach, the gastric fluids produced by the stomach cells must be used to store it, churn it, and blend it into a smooth mixture.

Upon completion of the pureeing process, the meal will go to the small intestine, where the bulk of the nutritional digestion will take place. It is responsible for the absorption of vitamins and minerals such as electrolytes, iron, carbohydrates, proteins, and fatty acids from the diet.

The remainder of the meal will next pass down to the large intestine, which will absorb the water component of the food and transport the wastes to the anus, where they will be expelled.

During this entire journey of food into the GI tract, all accessory organs of the digestive system, which includes the liver and pancreas, are also busy doing their purpose to complete the entire process.

Unfortunately, many people no longer have successful digestion that is free of complaints. In 2015, approximately 3 million adults in the United States were diagnosed with Inflammatory Bowel Disease (IBD) - a group of illnesses, including Crohn's disease, characterized by inflammation of the GI tract. It was previously thought to be an autoimmune disease. However, in line with recent studies, it is caused by the immune system fighting a harmless virus, bacterium, or food in the stomach, causing inflammation and intestinal damage as a result of the assault.

Still, there are ways to manage and prevent the progression of IBD. But, first and foremost, the following sections would delve deeper into the truths of IBD - its different types, risk factors, and truly effective preventive measures.

TYPES OF IBD, RISK FACTORS, AND PREVENTIVE MEASURES

What are the types of IBD?

There are two major types of IBD. These are ulcerative colitis and Crohn's disease.

- Ulcerative colitis only affects the innermost lining of the colon or large intestine, causing sores and swelling. What makes it distinct is that it does not skip or inflame any other parts of the colon, just the diseased section.
- Crohn's disease can affect any portion of the gastrointestinal tract. It usually affects the entire wall of the small intestine's terminal portion or the beginning of the colon. Also, in between areas of the diseased intestine, the inflammation skips or leaves unaffected portions.

Who is Affected?

IBD may affect individuals of any age, gender, or ethnicity and is not contagious. Despite the fact that the exact causes of the two types of IBD remain a mystery, researchers were able to uncover factors that were similar to all reported cases and which they think contribute to the higher risk of developing either of the two types of IBD.

According to studies, IBD is most often diagnosed in people between the ages of 15 and 35. Youngsters are twice as likely as adults to be diagnosed with Crohn's disease than with ulcerative colitis. In addition, it has been shown that males are somewhat more prone than females to suffer from IBD, according to research.

Many documented instances also demonstrate that heredity may play a role in developing IBD since most patients have first-degree relatives who are suffering from the disease before they too acquire the same condition. Cigarette smoking is also mentioned as one of the risk factors for IBD, as is having a family history of the disease. Active smokers have a twofold increased risk of developing ulcerative colitis or Crohn's disease compared to nonsmokers.

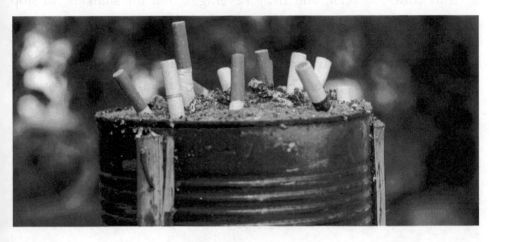

Furthermore, researchers discovered that Crohn's disease may afflict people of all racial origins, but that in recent years, the illness has grown more common among Caucasians, Hispanics, and Asians than in any other ethnic group. The use of nonsteroidal anti-inflammatory medicines (NSAIDs), birth control pills, and antibiotics has also been associated with an increased risk of Crohn's disease because of its effects on the gut wall.

Preventive Measures

As previously stated, the exact cause of IBD is not yet clear. However, there are still ways for you to reduce the risk of developing or worsening your IBD. The best method is to take extra care of yourself, which may be achieved by adopting a healthy diet.

Although it varies from case to case, your doctor may advise you to restrict the consumption of fiber and dairy products, to avoid certain beverages such as coffee, alcohol, and fizzy beverages, and for smokers, to stop smoking. This will depend on your specific circumstances. Aside from changing your meals, it is also important to complement them with regular activity and enough relaxation. These may assist you in maintaining your weight and managing stress, both of which can exacerbate digestive issues.

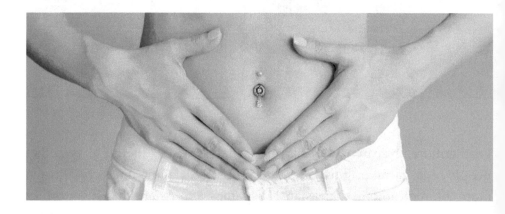

You may have to put in more effort to prevent the development of Crohn's if you already have a family history of the disease. It is important to know how the illness impacted your relatives in order to avoid developing it yourself.

CROHN'S DISEASE

Crohn's disease is a chronic condition that lasts a long time. Patients have frequent fluctuations in their symptoms, but they may go into remission at times. Patients' experiences are unique and vary from one another. Although the intensity of the symptoms may vary from minor to severe, it is possible that they will alter with time.

For patients with Crohn's, there are times of control (with few or no symptoms) as well as periods of active illness (with symptoms). The sooner you begin your treatment and management of the disease, the less probable it is for you to experience severe symptoms.

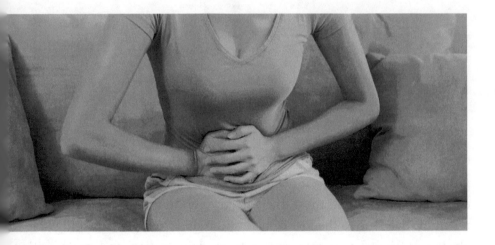

The symptoms of Crohn's disease may include diarrhea and stomach discomfort if the illness is mild to severe. You may not suffer any additional symptoms or problems, enabling you to go about your daily activities as normal, including walking, eating, and drinking. In general, the mild version of the illness has just a small impact on your day-to-day activities.

In addition to diarrhea or stomach discomfort, you may also experience other symptoms such as fever and anemia if you have moderate to severe Crohn's disease.

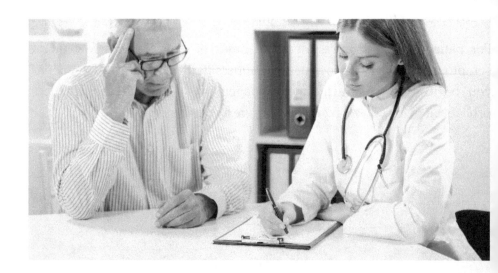

Crohn's disease is characterized by symptoms that have a major impact on your everyday life when it reaches its last or severe stage. You will be in constant pain and will most likely need to go to the toilet very often as a result of this. Due to the loss of body fluid and your gut not being able to absorb nutrients, you may suffer from dehydration and malnutrition. Because inflammation frequently occurs, almost nonstop, your bodily tissues are at greater risk of long-term damage.

Types of Crohn's Disease

While Crohn's disease symptoms differ from person to person, the type of Crohn's you have influences your symptoms and complications. Therefore, knowing which section of your GI tract is impacted is critical in determining what to expect. There are the following types of disease.

Ileocolitis

A form of Crohn's disease in which inflammation develops in the Ileum, the final part of the small intestine, and in the colon is called Ileocolitis. If you have this form of Crohn's disease, you may suffer from diarrhea, cramps, and discomfort on the right side of your abdomen. Also, be prepared for your body to drop weight all of a sudden.

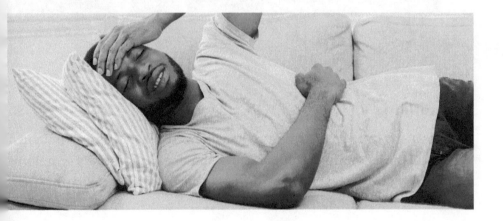

Ileitis

Ileitis, on the other hand, is a condition in which the Ileum is the only section of the intestine that is swollen and inflamed. In addition to the symptoms already listed above, severe cases may develop complications such as fistulas or an inflammatory abscess in the lower right abdomen.

Gastroduodenal

In case the inflammation and irritation impact both the stomach and the duodenum - the top part of the small intestine, you have developed Gastroduodenal. This type's symptoms include nausea, vomiting, loss of appetite, and significant weight loss.

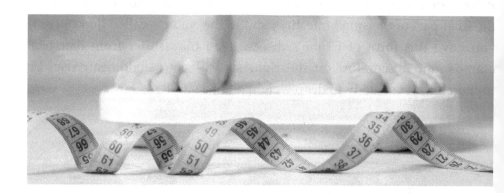

Jejunoileitis

Jejunoileitis is a type of Crohn's characterized by patches of inflamed sections of the Jejunum - the upper half of the small intestine. Its symptoms may include moderate to severe pain and cramps after meals, diarrhea, and for critical cases, formation of fistulas.

Crohn's Colitis

Crohn's colitis is the last type of Crohn's. It primarily affects the colon and causes diarrhea, rectal bleeding, skin lesions, joint pains, and abscesses, fistulas, or ulcers around the anus.

MANAGING THE SYMPTOMS

Crohn's disease patients could experience periods of flare-ups or serious symptoms followed by periods of remission or zero to moderate symptoms. The remission can last for weeks, months, or even years. Thus, it is impossible to predict when flare-ups will occur. But, how should one deal with Crohn's symptoms and complications as well as these fluctuations?

Crohn's disease management and treatment differ based on what is causing your symptoms and how severe they are. Given this, one or more of these Crohn's disease management methods and treatments may be recommended to you by your physician:

- **Antibiotics & Antidiarrheal Medications.** In order to cure the infection and avoid severe diarrhea, you might be recommended to take antibiotics and medicines such as loperamide to treat the infection and prevent severe diarrhea.
- **Bowel rest.** If you just had a flair, give your bowel time to rest. You should avoid solid, hard-to-chew meals and acidic beverages for several weeks in order to allow your intestines enough healing time. Choose well-cooked and easy-to-digest food, avoid alcohol, sugar, cigarettes, processed and fatty food. In severe cases, patients might get intravenous nourishment in order to obtain the necessary daily nutritional intake while also resting the bowel, relieving the stress and allowing them to recover more effectively.
- **Surgery.** Surgery does not cure Crohn's disease, but it can surely help with the complications. In severe cases, surgery may be required to repair intestinal holes, obstructions, or bleeding, which are all causing the illness to worsen.

- **Diet.** It is highly recommended that you consult with a registered dietician (RD) after visiting your doctor and confirming that you have Crohn's disease. An RD can help you understand how food might affect your symptoms and how eating a healthy diet can help you manage them. This would be quite beneficial in terms of managing your body weight and reducing the harmful impact food may have on your GI system.

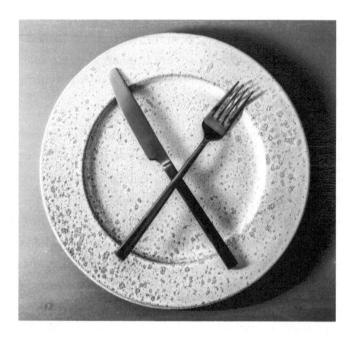

The following section will provide you with an idea of which foods to include in your meals.

CROHN'S DISEASE DIET

If you suffer from Crohn's disease, you should eat nutrient-dense foods. Your body requires the right nutrients to function optimally. They help the body to withstand appetite loss, weight loss and prevent malnutrition. Nutrient-dense foods improve an individual's well-being and can alleviate many experienced symptoms. On the other hand, meals high in calories but low in nutrients can worsen the condition—especially food which is spicy, fatty, sugary, or acidic.

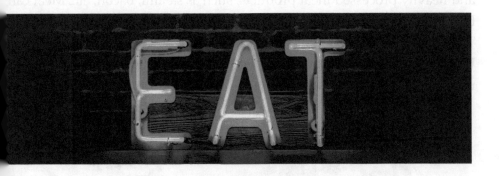

The effect of food differs from person to person. Individuals' eligibility for benefits is largely reliant on the kind of Crohn's disease they are suffering from, in addition to other criteria such as their age and gender.

As symptoms and severity of the disease vary from person to person, some types of food may work better for some patients while triggering the troubles for others. Therefore, it is critical to choose which meal plan is best for you. You may start by keeping note of your symptoms as you introduce or eliminate items from your diet. When in doubt about which foods to include or omit, you can follow our suggestions below.

Protein

Protein sources have been essential components of every dining and are significant to our body as protein maintains our cells, organs, and muscles to function properly and also helps guard our body against infections. It is essential to have a high-calorie, high-protein diet when suffering from Crohn's disease since nutrients are not easily absorbed. Choose protein sources that are low in fat, plant-based, and prepared in a way to make your digestion easier, if possible.

You are encouraged to eat lean protein sources such as poultry, lean fish and seafood and other types of lean meat. Stay away from fatty meat cuts and heavily processed meat products, such as salami, bacon, etc. Meat can be included in your meal plan if roasted, cooked, or baked without the skin. This method drains extra fat and ensures softness. Frying is not an option. Fried food is not only covered in fat and hard to digest, but it also isn't nutritious since many nutrients are lost during the preparation process.

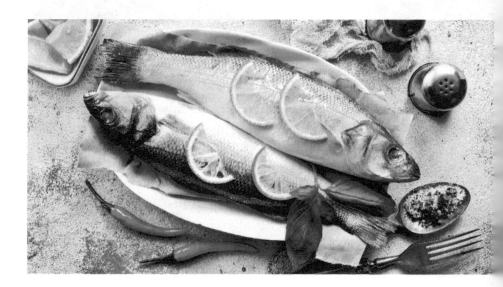

Seafood is also a great option because the meat is soft, does not include too much fat and has an excellent natural flavor, which does not need additional seasoning.

Another great protein source are eggs. Eggs are one of the healthiest and most nutrient-dense foods on the market. Many patients say that eggs are one of the most tolerable things to eat while suffering from Crohn's disease. However, make sure to cook your eggs thoroughly, as fresh eggs can cause a variety of digestive issues and may include dangerous bacteria. Avoid frying and over-seasoning.

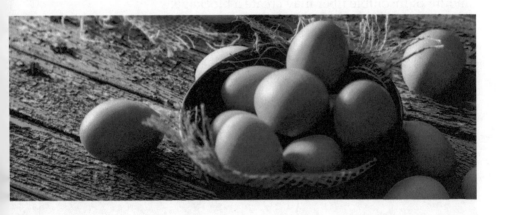

In addition, you can eat vegan protein sources, such as tofu and soy protein, as they include very little fat and are, in general, not irritating for your intestines.

Fiber

Consuming enough dietary fiber is beneficial to your overall health. It may assist you in maintaining appropriate levels of cholesterol, blood pressure, and body weight. Additionally, consuming about 23 grams of fiber each day may reduce your chance of experiencing a Crohn's flare by as much as 40%. However, while you are experiencing a flare, high-fiber meals may exacerbate your symptoms. It is, therefore, best to eat fibrous food during remission periods and avoid it once suffering from it.

If you suffer from Crohn's disease, foods that contain soluble fiber are the best option. Soluble fiber is a kind of fiber that absorbs excess fluid in the stomach and may aid in the slowing down of digestion and the alleviation of diarrhea. Insoluble fiber, on the other hand, has the potential to increase the quantity of water in your stomach. Watery diarrhea, stomach pains, and gas are all possible outcomes. In the worst-case scenario, an excessive amount of insoluble fiber may create a blockage.

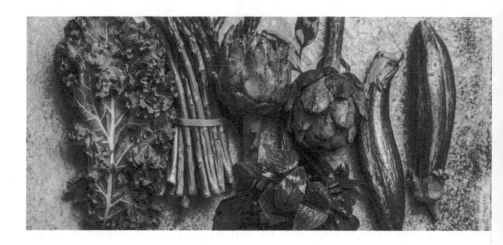

Foods derived from plants are the most nutritious sources of fiber. Fruits, vegetables, grains, beans, and nuts are all rich fiber sources. Among them, you should avoid nuts as they may worsen the inflammation in your intestines as well as your symptoms. Even though they include many healthy nutrients and healthy fats, they are hard to digest if eaten raw and unprocessed.

Another fibrous food group to avoid is whole grains, such as whole-grain bread, whole-wheat pasta, popcorn, and bran. They are hard to digest and may result in a significant quantity of movement in the gastrointestinal system, thus worsening your symptoms. Refined grains, on the other hand, have less fermentable fiber than whole grains, allowing them to move through the digestive system more rapidly than whole grains. They have a reputation for being gentler on the digestive system and less prone to induce inflammation. Examples of refined grains are white bread, pasta, white rice, etc.

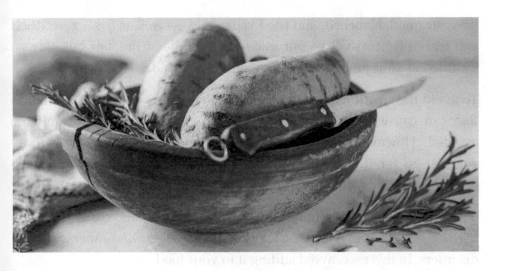

Among the fruit and vegetables, pick out the low fibrous ones. To reduce the amount of insoluble fiber they contain, you should remove their peels, skins, and seeds. You can also reduce the amount of fiber and make the vegetables and fruit easier to digest if you cook or puree them. Among the fruit, the best choices are apples (without the skin), peaches, honeydew melons, cantaloupes, watermelons and bananas. Among the vegetables, you are encouraged to consume pumpkins, squashes, cucumbers, bell peppers, beets, carrots, mushrooms, spinach, etc. Avocados, despite their increased fiber and fat content, may help you find malnourishment and can also be tolerated well for some people.

If you are experiencing severe symptoms or you're suffering from a flair, vegetables should be cooked until very soft, pureed, or juiced for faster consumption and absorption. Pureeing and mashing your food before serving reduces the amount of work the digestive system has to do, at least until your symptoms do not subside. Fruit should also be served in the form of purees or juices but have to be diluted in order to separate the pulp or fibers from the extracts.

Raw, steamed, blanched, and fried vegetables, as well as fresh, raw, dried and frozen fruits, shall be put aside for the time of the flair but may be included in your menu once your symptoms subside.

To avoid the creation of too much gas in the digestive system, vegetables that can cause it, such as cabbage, corn, and cauliflower, should be avoided. However, if you do not experience any troubles with those veggies, go for it. Everyone is different and some people might have difficulties eating certain types of food, while others don't.

Similarly, some people might be irritated by tomatoes and citrus fruits due to their acidity. It may cause them pain, acid reflux, and other digestive disorders. In this case, avoid adding it to your food.

Also, look for additional fiber in meals you wouldn't anticipate, such as dairy products, by reading the labels.

Fat

Crohn's disease may cause your body's capacity to digest and absorb fat to be impaired. The undigested fat will pass through your small intestine and into your colon, resulting in diarrhea and constipation. The consumption of larger quantities of unhealthy fat (reach in omega-six fatty acids) over long periods of time may cause chronic inflammation in your intestines as well as high cholesterol levels and thus worsen your symptoms. As a result, you should avoid highly refined fat sources, fried and greasy foods, processed food, as it is covered in oil, mayonnaise, margarine and other unhealthy fatty sauces, as much as possible.

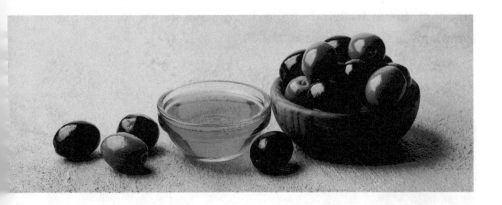

On the other hand, new studies suggest that eating healthy fat may help to decrease the bacteria in the gut and, as a result, may help to lessen the detrimental inflammation that Crohn's disease patients suffer. Healthy fat sources are high in omega-three fatty acids and have anti-inflammatory qualities. Healthy fat sources, including plant-based and cold-pressed oils such as olive oil or and avocado oil, may help you fulfill your daily fat need by providing you with the necessary nutrients. Healthy fat can also be obtained through fish, meat, eggs and avocados.

Dairy and Probiotics

You can have up to 2 kilograms of bacteria in your digestive system. These clusters of bacteria are called your microbiome, a type of bacterial fingerprint that is unique to you. If you have Crohn's disease, the balance between good and bad bacteria can be destroyed. Restoring the balance can help improve your symptoms. Probiotics are healthy bacteria that are found in the food you eat or enter your body with nutritional supplements. They can help improve the symptoms of bowel inflammation and digestion. Some bacterial strains have been shown to help reduce the symptoms of Crohn's disease.

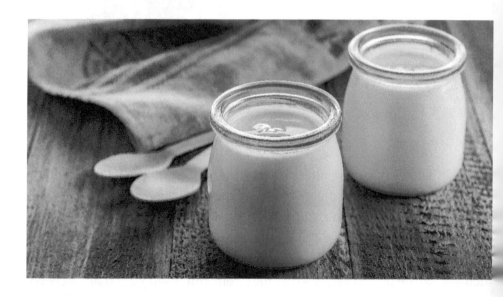

It is best to focus on the right food sources first, as these also contain other nutrients, but also because the quality of nutritional supplements can vary. Dietary sources of probiotics include:

- Yogurt (if you are sensitive to dairy products, avoid it)

- Kombucha
- Kimchi
- Kefir
- Cucumbers
- Tofu

As for the other dairy products, some people may benefit from hard cheeses like Cheddar and Parmesan since they contain less lactose. Lactose is a milk sugar that may cause discomfort and bloating. In addition, goat milk and dairy products, made from goat milk, contain almost no lactose, so it may be a great addition to one's meals while on a Crohn's disease diet.

However, some patients may suffer severe lactose intolerance and have trouble digesting all types of dairy products as it may cause them an upset stomach, abdominal cramps, and diarrhea. If you have such symptoms, omit the animal-sourced diary from your menu completely or pick out vegan types and lactose-free dairy products.

Drinks

Crohn's disease can cause diarrhea and bleeding and can affect your body's ability to absorb water from your digestive tract, which could lead to dehydration. Research indicates that liquids or liquid diets may be beneficial for individuals suffering from Crohn's disease, especially during a flare-up of their condition. The liquid diet, which allows the intestines to take a much-needed break, may help to reduce the symptoms of Crohn's disease. In addition, the liquid diet or specific high-calorie liquid formulations may benefit individuals with Crohn's disease who need additional nourishment for a short period of time or whose intestines are unable to absorb adequate nutrients from traditional meals.

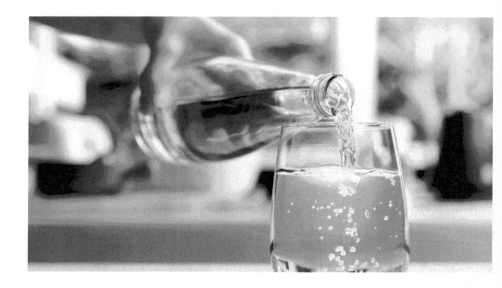

So, make it a habit to drink 8 to 10 glasses of water daily. As for the liquid diet, go for the pureed, well-cooked vegetable soups and smoothies. You can also try the following teas, which are known to have anti-inflammatory and healing properties, and they might help flush toxins out of the body:

- Ginger tea
- Green tea
- Mint tea
- Chamomile tea
- Curcumin tea

In addition, add to your diet natural vegetable and fruit juices without pulp. They won't only rehydrate you but also provide you with the necessary vitamins and minerals that your body needs to function normally.

Caffeinated, cream-based, sugary and alcoholic beverages should be avoided as they trigger irritations and may worsen your symptoms.

Food Preparation and Meal Planning

It is not only important to pick out the right type of food for yourself, but the preparation and planning of your meals matter as well. Here are some practices to consider when preparing and planning your meals.

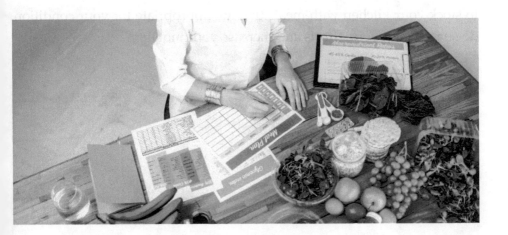

- **Eat in Small Servings**

It is advised to eat food between 4-6 times each day. As a matter of fact, eating smaller portions of food many times a day is preferable to eating bigger portions twice or three times daily. Smaller meal portions make it easier for the gastrointestinal system to digest and absorb the nutrients from the food you consume.

- **Stay Hydrated**

Make it a habit to consume enough water to keep your urine light yellow or clear and your body hydrated throughout the day. You may also want to consider consuming broth, vegetable juice, tea and other natural rehydration beverages without added sugar to keep your body fluids in balance.

- **Plan and Stock**

Plan, prepare and divide the meals you want to eat during the day, as well as the meals you intend to have the next day if at all feasible. If you are able to stock your kitchen with meals that are appropriate for your condition, do so to reduce your efforts and increase your mobility.

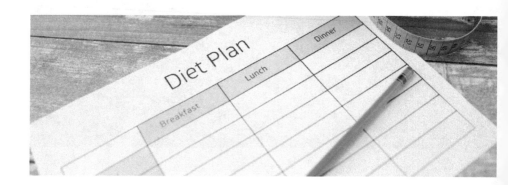

- **Keep it Simple**

You should get familiar with basic culinary methods such as boiling, grilling, and steaming. These methods are simple to learn, do not take a lot of time and help to preserve the nutrients in the food which you are preparing, as well as making it easier to digest.

- **Keep a Journal**

It is strongly suggested that you maintain a diary for every diet and condition you are following so that you can track your food consumption as well as any new symptoms you may be experiencing at any time. As a result, both you and your physician will have a better knowledge of your situation. You may utilize this information to better plan your meals and therapies in order to preserve your body's health.

- **Consult with a Dietitian**

Before drastically changing your diet, you should consult with your doctor or a registered dietitian to determine what are the best options for you and your specific needs, symptoms, and current condition.

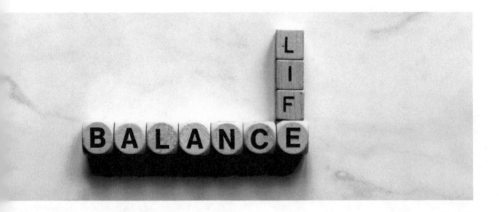

On the following pages, you can find 60 healthy and easy-to-make recipes. The recipes are divided into 3 chapters and tailored for the Crohn's disease diet. After reading the next pages, you will learn how to make delicious meals, as well as learn some preparation tricks and food facts. At the end of the book, there is a 2-week diet plan to help you transition to your diet.

So, let's not waste any more time. Grab your apron and let's head into the kitchen

BREAKFAST

Potato & Spinach Frittata

Prep time: 20 min	Cook time: 30 min	Servings: 2

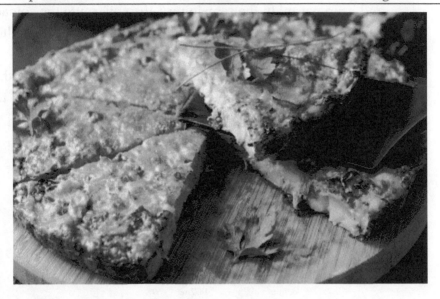

Ingredients

- _3 eggs_
- _½ cup yogurt_
- _1 tsp kosher salt_
- _1 cup potatoes, cut into small pieces_
- _2 tbsp olive oil_
- _1 cup chopped spinach_
- _¼ small red onion, chopped_
- _1 tsp garlic powder_
- _1 oz. goat cheese_

Directions

- Preheat the oven to 350 ° F.
- Combine eggs, yogurt and salt in a mixing bowl.
- In a 10-inch ovenproof nonstick skillet, sauté potatoes in 1 tbsp heated oil for 8 to 10 minutes, or until soft and golden; remove and keep warm. In the remaining 1 tbsp oil, sauté the spinach and onion for about 3 to 4 minutes, or until spinach is wilted and tender. Mix in potatoes.
- Pour the egg mixture over the vegetables and cook for another 3 minutes. After it is done, sprinkle the goat cheese over the vegetable and put it in the oven.
- Bake for 10 to 14 minutes, or until set.

NUTRITION FACTS (PER SERVING)

Calories	338	
Total Fat	20.2g	26%
Saturated Fat	12.3g	62%
Cholesterol	298mg	99%
Sodium	1377mg	60%
Total Carbohydrate	19.4g	7%
Dietary Fiber	2.5g	9%
Total Sugars	6.8g	
Protein	19.3g	

Tips: In order to avoid too much air entering the mixture, just beat the eggs until they are barely combined. As the frittata bakes, the eggs will continue to swell and puff up. This may result in a spongy, dry, and unpleasant feel on the surface.

Beet and Kiwi Smoothie

| Prep time: 10 min | Cook time: 0 min | Servings: 2 |

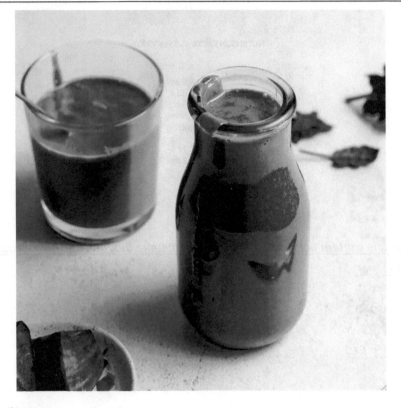

Ingredients

- *1 red beet, cooked, peeled and cubed*
- *1 kiwi, peeled and cubed*
- *a handful of coriander*
- *1 cup water*

Directions

- Add all ingredients into a blender.
- Blend until smooth and creamy.
- Pour into glasses and enjoy.

NUTRITION FACTS (PER SERVING)

Calories	91	
Total Fat	0.6g	1%
Saturated Fat	0.1g	0%
Cholesterol	0mg	0%
Sodium	88mg	4%
Total Carbohydrate	21.3g	8%
Dietary Fiber	4.4g	16%
Total Sugars	14.8g	
Protein	2.6g	

Tips: Kiwis contain actinidin, a proteolytic enzyme that aids in the breakdown of proteins.

Beet Hash

| Prep time: 10 min | Cook time: 20 min | Servings: 2 |

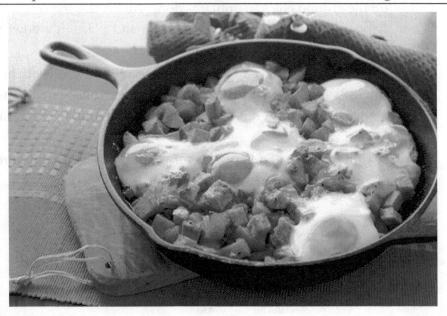

Ingredients

- 2 large beets
- 3 tbsp vegetable oil
- ½ bell pepper chopped
- ½ lb. chicken, ground
- ¼ cup leek, chopped
- ½ cup carrot
- salt and black pepper
- 2 tbsp freshly chopped basil

Directions

- Microwave beets until they are cooked but not mushy. Peel the beets and chop them into little cubes.
- In a large skillet, heat 2 tbsp oil over medium-high heat and add bell pepper and carrot. Cook until the vegetables are soft. Break up the ground chicken until it is done. Add leeks, then cook for 1 more minute. Remove from the pan and place in a bowl to cool.
- In the same skillet, add the remaining oil and the beets in a single layer. Allow to cook for 5 minutes (uncovered) until golden brown, then mix and continue to boil until the beets are golden.
- Season with salt and pepper before adding the turkey mixture.
- Garnish with basil. If desired, put one or two fried eggs on top!

NUTRITION FACTS (PER SERVING)

Calories	398	
Total Fat	22.8g	29%
Saturated Fat	4.6g	23%
Cholesterol	63mg	21%
Sodium	132mg	6%
Total Carbohydrate	21g	8%
Dietary Fiber	3.9g	14%
Total Sugars	6.8g	
Protein	29g	

Tips: Beetroots provide substantial volumes of manganese, potassium, iron, and vitamin C, plus fiber, folate and other minerals. Beetroot and beet juice provide a number of health benefits, including enhanced blood flow and reduced blood pressure.

Banana Protein Smoothie

Prep time: 5 min	Cook time: 0 min	Servings: 4

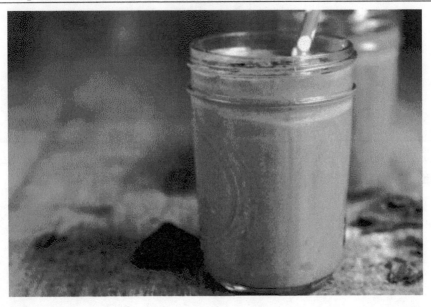

Ingredients

- 1 banana, frozen
- 1 scoop vanilla protein powder
- ½ cup low-fat coconut milk
- 2 tsp unsweetened cocoa powder

Directions

- In a blender, combine banana, milk, vanilla protein powder, cocoa powder and honey.
- Cover and blend until smooth.

NUTRITION FACTS (PER SERVING)

Calories	307	
Total Fat	3.5g	4%
Saturated Fat	2g	10%
Cholesterol	12mg	4%
Sodium	113mg	5%
Total Carbohydrate	41.2g	15%
Dietary Fiber	4.8g	17%
Total Sugars	26g	
Protein	33g	

Tips: Bananas are also loaded with calcium, magnesium, zinc, and vitamins A, B6, B12, fiber, and folic acid, which are essential vitamins and nutrients that help babies gain a healthy weight.

Scrambled Eggs

Prep time: 5 min	Cook time: 5 min	Servings: 2

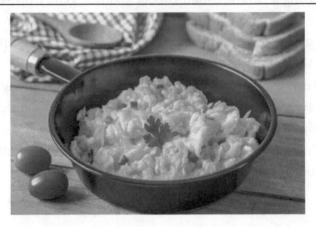

Ingredients

- 4 large eggs
- ¼ cup coconut milk
- salt, to taste
- fresh herbs to taste (parsley, basil…)
- 1 tbsp olive oil

Directions

- Crack the eggs into a glass bowl and beat them until they turn light yellow.
- Add the milk to the eggs and season with salt and fresh herbs. Beat the eggs like crazy. If you're not up to it, you can use an electric mixer or a stand mixer with a whisk. Whichever device you use, try to get as much air as possible into the eggs.

- Preheat a solid-bottomed nonstick skillet over medium-low heat. Add the oil and let it melt.
- When the saucepan is hot enough, pour the eggs into it. Do not stir. Let the eggs cook for up to a minute or until the bottom hardens but does not brown.
- Using a heat-resistant rubber spatula, gently press on the edge of the egg toward the center while tilting the pan to allow the egg, which is still liquid, to sink underneath. Repeat with the other edges until all of the liquid is gone.
- Turn off the heat and keep stirring the egg gently until all the raw parts are firm. Do not break the egg and keep the curd as big as possible. As you add more ingredients, add them quickly.
- Transfer to a plate when the eggs are ready but still moist and soft. Serve immediately and enjoy.

NUTRITION FACTS (PER SERVING)

Calories	329	
Total Fat	30.7g	39%
Saturated Fat	21.2g	106%
Cholesterol	372mg	124%
Sodium	222mg	10%
Total Carbohydrate	2.5g	1%
Dietary Fiber	0.7g	2%
Total Sugars	1.8g	
Protein	13.3g	

Tips: Make it easy on yourself and cook your eggs in a nonstick sauté pan. Use a heat-resistant silicone spatula so it doesn't melt or scratch the pan.

Melon Smoothie

Prep time: 10 min	Cook time: 0 min	Servings: 2

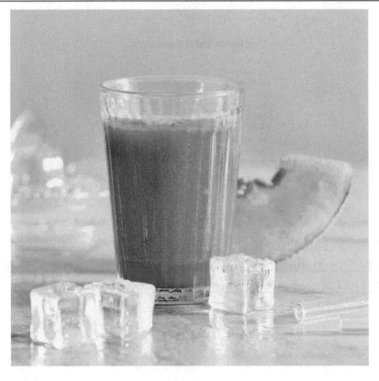

Ingredients

- ⅛ melon, peeled, seeded and cubed
- ¼ cup green grapes, peeled, seeded and cubed
- 1 apple, peeled, seeded and cubed
- 1 tbsp honey

Directions

- Add all ingredients into a blender.
- Blend until smooth and creamy.
- Pour into glasses and enjoy.

NUTRITION FACTS (PER SERVING)		
Calories	72	
Total Fat	0.3g	0%
Saturated Fat	0g	0%
Cholesterol	0mg	0%
Sodium	6mg	0%
Total Carbohydrate	18.4g	7%
Dietary Fiber	1.5g	5%
Total Sugars	16.1g	
Protein	0.8g	

Tips: Melons are well tolerated by Crohn's disease patients. They can be eaten raw, as they are easy to digest. In addition, they include many vitamins, including vitamins A and C, and are a very strong antioxidants.

Avocado and Oatmeal Smoothie

Prep time: 5 min	Cook time: 0 min	Servings: 2

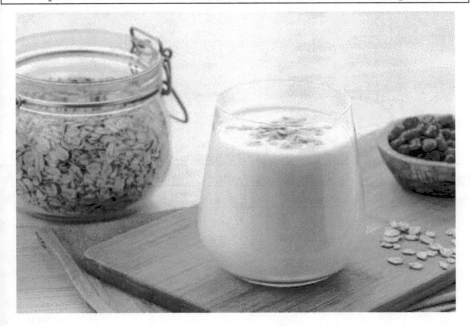

Ingredients

- *1 cup soy milk*
- *1 large avocado*
- *½ cup oatmeal*
- *1 tsp vanilla extract*
- *4 ice cubes*

Directions

- Add all ingredients into a blender.
- Blend until smooth and creamy.

- Pour into glasses and enjoy.

NUTRITION FACTS (PER SERVING)

Calories	251	
Total Fat	5.3g	7%
Saturated Fat	0.7g	3%
Cholesterol	0mg	0%
Sodium	219mg	10%
Total Carbohydrate	47.4g	17%
Dietary Fiber	6.6g	24%
Total Sugars	17.4g	
Protein	5.2g	

Tips: Avocados are high in heart-healthy monounsaturated fat, which can help battle malnutrition. Avocados, which are nutrient- and calorie-dense, can help you fuel your body in a healthy way if you're losing weight due to Crohn's disease.

Breakfast Muffins

Prep time: 5 min	Cook time: 20 min	Servings: 2

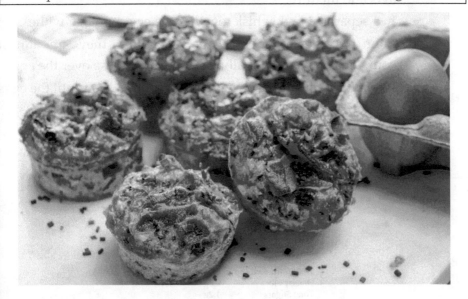

Ingredients

- ⅜ *cup cherry tomatoes, chopped*
- ½ *cup fresh kale leaves, chopped*
- ½ *avocado, seeded, peeled and diced*
- *salt and pepper, to taste*
- *1 egg*
- ¼ *cup egg whites*
- ½ *tbsp crumbled goat cheese*

Directions

- Preheat the oven to 350 ° F.

- Coat a normal nonstick mini muffin tray with a cooking spray or parchment paper.
- Combine tomatoes, spinach, avocado, salt and pepper in a medium-sized mixing bowl.
- Fill each tiny muffin cup with two tbsp of the veggie and avocado mixture.
- In a separate bowl, whisk together the eggs and egg whites.
- Pour the eggs over the vegetables until they are almost completely covered. Finally, sprinkle the cheese over the eggs.
- Put in the oven and bake for about 20 minutes, or until the eggs bounce back when pressed.

NUTRITION FACTS (PER SERVING)

Calories	110	
Total Fat	7.8g	10%
Saturated Fat	1.7g	8%
Cholesterol	76mg	25%
Sodium	113mg	5%
Total Carbohydrate	4.7g	2%
Dietary Fiber	2.8g	10%
Total Sugars	1.2g	
Protein	25.5g	

Tips: In addition to a range of nutrients such as vitamins, minerals, and fiber, kale includes a variety of phytochemicals that are beneficial to everyone, including individuals who have Crohn's disease. Unfortunately, kale may be difficult to digest; therefore, you should eat it fresh only when in remission. Otherwise, remember to cook it well prior to consuming it.

Easy Oatmeal Pancakes

| Prep time: 15 min | Cook time: 20 min | Servings: 2 |

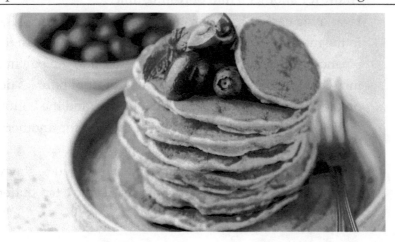

Ingredients

- ½ cup old-fashioned rolled oats
- ½ cup almond milk
- ½ tbsp unsalted butter, plus more for cooking
- 1 large egg
- ½ tbsp applesauce
- ⅓ cup almond flour
- 2 tsp baking powder
- ¼ tsp kosher salt
- ¼ tsp ground nutmeg (optional)

Directions

- In a large mixing bowl, combine rolled oats and almond milk.

- Allow 10 min for the oats to soften. In the meantime, melt 1 tbsp of unsalted butter in a small saucepan and leave it aside to cool.
- Combine the oats with the butter, 1 egg, and ½ tbsp apple sauce and mix to blend. Whisk together almond flour, baking powder, kosher salt, and ground nutmeg. Do not overmix. Allow for another 5 min of resting time.
- Heat a big cast iron or nonstick skillet over medium-high heat in the meantime. Swirl 1 tsp butter into the pan to coat it. Cook 3 pancakes at a time, dropping the batter into the pan in 2-tbsp increments. Cook for about 3 minutes, or until bubbles develop on the surface, the edges begin to look dry, and the bottoms are golden brown. Flip the pancakes and cook for another 2 to 3 minutes, or until golden brown on the other side.
- Place the pancakes on a dish or in a heated oven to stay warm. Cook the remaining batter in batches, using 1 tsp butter each time.

NUTRITION FACTS (PER SERVING)

Calories	277	
Total Fat	8.6g	11%
Saturated Fat	3.6g	18%
Cholesterol	106mg	35%
Sodium	234mg	10%
Total Carbohydrate	39.4g	14%
Dietary Fiber	3.2g	11%
Total Sugars	6.5g	
Protein	10.8g	

Tips: The pancakes can be refrigerated for up to 5 days or frozen for up to 2 months if stored in an airtight container.

Sweet Potato Flounder Frittata

Prep time: 15 min	Cook time: 25 min	Servings: 2

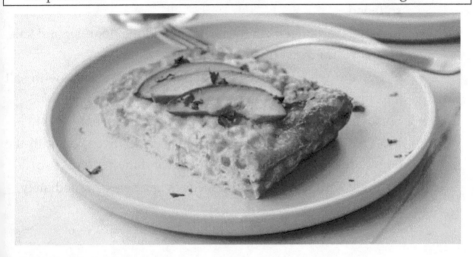

Ingredients

- 1 tbsp olive oil
- 1 small potato, peeled and cut into 1" cubes
- ½ Anaheim peppers thinly sliced
- ½ celery, trimmed and thinly sliced
- ¾ cups cooked flounder separated into chunks
- ¾ cups fresh kale leaves
- ½ cup grated goat cheese optional
- 3 large eggs beaten just until whites and yolks are combined
- ½ tsp salt
- ½ tsp pepper
- ¼ cup chopped basil

49

Directions

- Preheat the oven to 350 ° F. In a 10" oven-safe skillet, such as cast iron, heat the oil over medium-high heat. Add potatoes.
- Cook, tossing frequently until the potato cubes are soft and slightly crunchy. Add celery and peppers and cook until softened.
- Remove the skillet from the heat and add the flounder and kale, arranging them evenly in the pan.
- Crack and wish the eggs in a separate bowl, season with salt and pepper. Pour them over the skillet's contents.
- Sprinkle over the cheese (if using). Put in the oven.
- Bake for 15-20 minutes in the center of the oven, or until the edges are peeling away from the pan and the center is set.
- Sprinkle with basil, slice into wedges and serve immediately.

NUTRITION FACTS (PER SERVING)

Calories	332	
Total Fat	18.8g	24%
Saturated Fat	7.3g	37%
Cholesterol	61mg	20%
Sodium	597mg	26%
Total Carbohydrate	15.9g	6%
Dietary Fiber	2.6g	9%
Total Sugars	4.2g	
Protein	26.4g	

Tips: The high-fiber potato skins should be avoided since they are likely to cause inflammation, but the insides of potatoes can be beneficial to eat for Crohn's disease patients. Potatoes, like bananas, are high in potassium and can assist your body to maintain its fluid balance while you're dealing with a flare-up.

Sweet Potato Pancakes

| Prep time: 5 min | Cook time: 20 min | Servings: 4 |

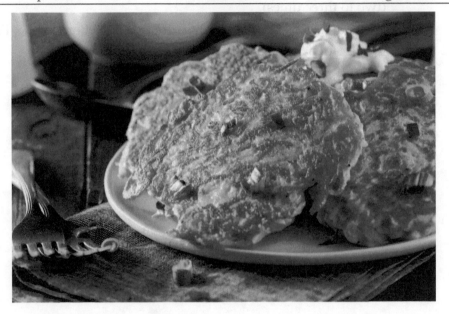

Ingredients

- 1 large sweet potato, peeled and cubed (about 1 cup), divided
- ½ medium onion, cubed
- 1 large egg
- 1-½ tbsp soy flour
- 1 tbsp minced fresh dill
- ¼ tsp baking powder
- ½ tsp salt and pepper
- ⅛ tsp ground cinnamon

Directions

- Add ½ a cup of sweet potatoes, onion, 1 egg, flour, dill, baking powder, salt, pepper, and cinnamon in a blender or food processor. Blend until completely smooth.
- Pulse in the remaining potatoes until they are finely minced (two to three times).
- ¼ cup at a time, pour over a hot, greased skillet or griddle. Fry until golden brown on both sides, over medium heat.

NUTRITION FACTS (PER SERVING)

Calories	99	
Total Fat	1.4g	2%
Saturated Fat	0.4g	2%
Cholesterol	47mg	16%
Sodium	174mg	8%
Total Carbohydrate	18.4g	7%
Dietary Fiber	2.7g	10%
Total Sugars	1.8g	
Protein	3.6g	

Tips: During a Crohn's flare-up, sweet potatoes can be lifesavers. They include many vitamins and minerals and are, if cooked well, easy to digest. Just stay away from the potato peels, which may cause digestive problems.

Pork, Sweet Potato & Egg Bake

| Prep time: 5 min | Cook time: 20 min | Servings: 4 |

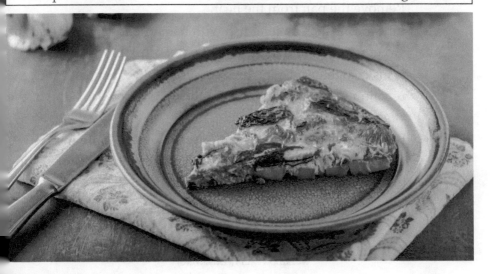

Ingredients

- ½ pound lean ground pork (90% lean)
- ½ cup chopped onion
- 1 tsp salt, divided
- 1 tsp garlic, minced
- ¼ tsp rubbed dill
- 1 cup chopped kale
- 1 cup frozen shredded hash brown sweet potatoes
- 4 eggs
- ⅓ cup goat cheese
- ⅓ cup soymilk
- ½ cup shredded feta cheese

53

Directions

- Preheat the oven to 350 ° F. Cook pork, onion, ½ tsp of salt, minced garlic and dill in a large skillet over medium heat for 6-8 minutes, or until the pork is no longer pink.
- Drain the extra fat from the skillet. Add the kale and mix well. Remove the pan from the heat.
- Line a 13x9-inch baking dish with parchment paper, spread the sweet potatoes and top it with the pork mixture.
- Whisk together eggs, goat cheese, milk, pepper, and the remaining salt in a large mixing bowl; pour over the top of the vegetables and pork.
- Bake uncovered for 45-50 minutes, or until a knife inserted in the center comes out clean Allow for 5-10 minutes of resting time before serving.

NUTRITION FACTS (PER SERVING)

Calories	267	
Total Fat	14.5g	19%
Saturated Fat	5.5g	27%
Cholesterol	264mg	88%
Sodium	492mg	21%
Total Carbohydrate	9.1g	3%
Dietary Fiber	1.5g	5%
Total Sugars	1.6g	
Protein	24.3g	

Tips: Eggs are an excellent, low-cost source of protein. Egg whites include more than half of the protein in an egg, as well as vitamin B2 and less fat than the yolk Selenium, vitamins D, B6, and B12, as well as minerals including zinc, iron, and copper, are abundant in eggs.

Sweet Potato Omelette

Prep time: 5 min	Cook time: 20 min	Servings: 2

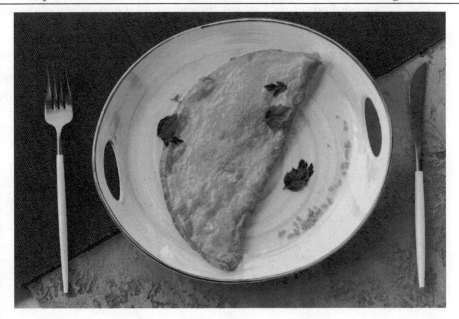

Ingredients

- 1 tbsp butter
- 6 eggs
- 4 tbsp onion powder
- ⅛ tsp salt
- freshly ground black pepper to taste
- 1 cup cubed cooked sweet potato
- ¼ cup shredded goat cheese

Directions

- Melt the butter in a skillet over medium-high heat. Combine the eggs, onion powder, water, salt, and pepper in a mixing bowl. Pour the egg mixture into the skillet (mixture should set immediately at the edges).
- Push cooked edges toward the center as the eggs set, allowing the uncooked portion to flow below.
- Once the eggs have set, add sweet potato cubes over one side of the eggs and top with cheese; fold the other side over the filling. Arrange the omelette on a plate. If desired, sprinkle with freshly chopped herbs, such as basil or parsley.

NUTRITION FACTS (PER SERVING)

Calories	481	
Total Fat	34.1g	44%
Saturated Fat	17.4g	87%
Cholesterol	551mg	184%
Sodium	738mg	32%
Total Carbohydrate	19.1g	7%
Dietary Fiber	1.9g	7%
Total Sugars	2.7g	
Protein	25.5g	

Tips: Despite the vast lists of foods to avoid, there are still plenty of delicious brunch options if you have Crohn's disease. Eggs are a good source of lean protein. Scrambled eggs, quiche, and frittatas are among our suggestions.

Acorn Squash Breakfast Bowl

| Prep time: 5 min | Cook time: 20 min | Servings: 2 |

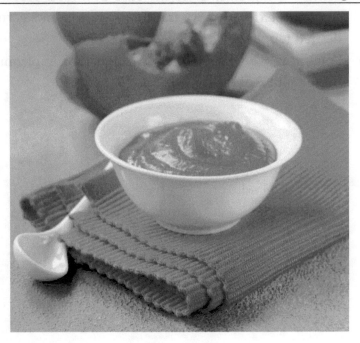

Ingredients

Base

- *½ large acorn squash, cooked*
- *⅛ cup almond milk*
- *1 tsp vanilla optional*

Toppings

- *2 bananas, sliced*

- *1-2 cups melon*
- *¼ cup kiwi*
- *pumpkin pie spice to taste*

Directions

- Blend the ingredients for the base in a food processor until smooth. Before serving, transfer to bowls and garnish with desired toppings.
- Squash can be stored in the fridge for simple meal prep throughout the week!

NUTRITION FACTS (PER SERVING)

Calories	178	
Total Fat	7.9g	10%
Saturated Fat	4g	20%
Cholesterol	0mg	0%
Sodium	6mg	0%
Total Carbohydrate	27.3g	10%
Dietary Fiber	4g	14%
Total Sugars	13.3g	
Protein	3.8g	

Tips: Acorn squash has a variety of nutrients, including fiber, vitamin C, potassium, and magnesium, among others. It also contains many useful plant components, such as carotenoid antioxidants, which are powerful antioxidants. Therefore, acorn squash may be beneficial for general health and may help to guard against some chronic diseases such as heart disease and type 2 diabetes.

Carrot Muffins

| Prep time: 20 min | Cook time: 20 min | Servings: 12 |

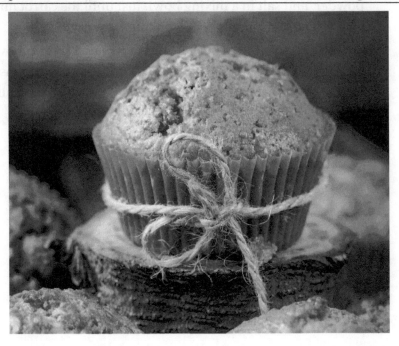

Ingredients

- 1-pound carrots, peeled and cut into 1-inch slices
- ½ cup butter, melted
- 1 large egg, lightly beaten
- 1-½ cups soy flour
- ½ cup maple syrup
- 2-½ tsp baking powder
- ½ tsp salt

Directions

- In a saucepan, add 1 inch of water and the carrot. Bring the water to a boil. Reduce heat to low, cover, and cook for 5 minutes, or until vegetables are soft. Drain and mash, then add the butter and egg. Combine the flour, maple syrup, baking powder, and salt in a mixing bowl. Just until the carrot mixture is moistened, stir in the remaining ingredients.
- Fill muffin cups three-quarters full with batter. Preheat oven to 375°F and bake for 20-25 minutes, or until a toothpick inserted in the middle comes out clean. Allow to cool for 5 minutes before transferring to a wire rack.

NUTRITION FACTS (PER SERVING)

Calories	150	
Total Fat	8.3g	11%
Saturated Fat	5g	25%
Cholesterol	36mg	12%
Sodium	162mg	7%
Total Carbohydrate	18g	7%
Dietary Fiber	0.7g	3%
Total Sugars	9.1g	
Protein	2.1g	

Tips: Carrots are nutrient-dense and contain antioxidants that help treat Crohn's disease. Peeled and cooked carrots are also a lot easier to digest than raw carrots. To assist your body, keep its fluids balanced, avoid the fiber-rich peels and enjoy the potassium-rich, mushy insides of potatoes.

Tofu and Egg Muffins

Prep time: 20 min	Cook time: 20 min	Servings: 12

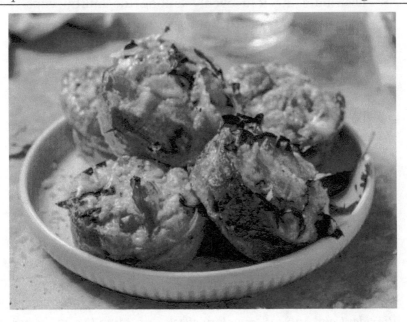

Ingredients

- *10 large eggs*
- *1 tsp sea salt and black pepper or to taste*
- *½ tsp garlic, minced*
- *⅓ cup chopped chives*
- *1 cup tofu, chopped and cooked*

Directions

- Preheat the oven to 400 ° F.

- Use silicone liners or nonstick cooking spray to line a 12-count muffin pan.
- Crack eggs into a large measuring cup or mixing bowl and stir with salt, black pepper and garlic. Add chives.
- Fill each muffin cup about ⅔ full with the mixture.
- Distribute the tofu evenly among the muffin cups using a spoon. Bake for 12-16 minutes, or until set, in a preheated oven.

NUTRITION FACTS (PER SERVING)

Calories	74	
Total Fat	4.2g	5%
Saturated Fat	1.3g	6%
Cholesterol	164mg	55%
Sodium	102mg	4%
Total Carbohydrate	0.9g	0%
Dietary Fiber	0.1g	0%
Total Sugars	0.4g	
Protein	8.2g	

Tips: Soy and tofu, in addition to lean protein, include bioactive peptides, which have antioxidant and anti-inflammatory effects, according to some research, and may help control Crohn's disease.

Easy Quiche

| Prep time: 15 min | Cook time: 25 min | Servings: 2 |

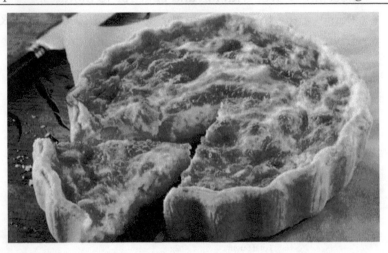

Ingredients

- 1 tbsp butter
- ¼ cup onion diced
- ⅓ lb. zucchini, peeled and diced
- 1 cup cooked tempeh
- 3 large eggs
- 1 ¼ cups grated feta cheese
- 3 tbsp soy milk
- salt & pepper to taste
- 10-inch tart shell, unbaked

Directions

- Preheat the oven to 375 ° F.

- Melt the butter in a small skillet and cook the onion until soft and faintly browned, about 5 minutes.
- Place sautéed onions, diced tempeh, half of the cheese, eggs, milk, salt, and pepper in a large mixing bowl. Stir. Pour the mixture into the tart shell. Finish with the remaining cheese and zucchini. Cover with foil and bake for 15 minutes.
- Remove the foil and bake for another 5-10 minutes. Remove from the oven and set aside for 10 minutes to cool before serving.

NUTRITION FACTS (PER SERVING)

Calories	347	
Total Fat	23.3g	30%
Saturated Fat	6.3g	31%
Cholesterol	163mg	54%
Sodium	159mg	7%
Total Carbohydrate	5.4g	2%
Dietary Fiber	1.4g	5%
Total Sugars	2g	
Protein	10.4g	

Tips: Any type of squash or vegetable, in general, is best tolerated for Crohn's patients when peeled and well cooked. Try not to eat raw vegetables too often, especially if you are experiencing a flair.

Tempeh Pancakes

Prep time: 10 min	Cook time: 10 min	Servings: 4

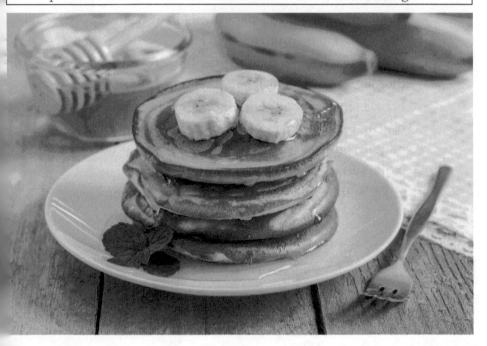

Ingredients

- ½ pack tempeh
- 1 tsp vanilla extract
- 1 cup coconut milk
- ½ tbsp olive oil
- ½ almond flour
- 2 tbsp maple syrup
- ½ tsp ground cardamom

- ½ tbsp baking powder
- ½ tsp salt

Directions

- Blend tempeh, vanilla, and milk in a large mixing bowl until a thick batter forms.
- Combine all of the dry ingredients in a separate bowl, making sure there are no lumps.
- Pour the tempeh mixture into the dry ingredients and stir thoroughly until a thick batter with no lumps forms.
- Pour a small amount of oil into a big nonstick frying pan and heat it up. Pour pancake batter onto a pan and cook for 2 minutes on each side, or until bubbles appear over the majority of the surface.
- Enjoy with maple syrup and freshly cut bananas.

NUTRITION FACTS (PER SERVING)

Calories	492	
Total Fat	39.9g	51%
Saturated Fat	27.2g	136%
Cholesterol	0mg	0%
Sodium	611mg	27%
Total Carbohydrate	27.8g	10%
Dietary Fiber	3.6g	13%
Total Sugars	16.2g	
Protein	12g	

Tips: Tempeh is particularly high in helpful prebiotics. According to research, tempeh was found to promote the growth of Bifidobacterium, a species of good gut bacteria.

Honeydew Smoothie

Prep time: 5 min	Cook time: 0 min	Servings: 1

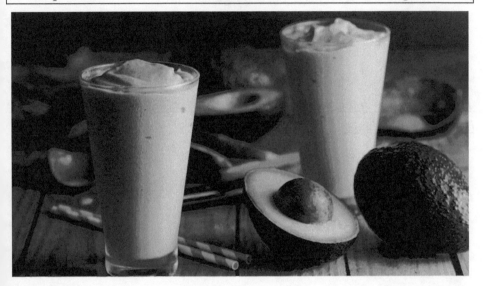

Ingredients

- 1 cup diced honeydew
- ½ avocado
- ½ cup coconut milk
- 1 tbsp chia seeds
- ½ tsp maple syrup

Directions

- Put all the ingredients in a blender.
- Blend until smooth.
- Serve immediately and enjoy!

NUTRITION FACTS (PER SERVING)

Calories	289	
Total Fat	5.6g	7%
Saturated Fat	1g	5%
Cholesterol	0mg	0%
Sodium	76mg	3%
Total Carbohydrate	60.5g	22%
Dietary Fiber	5.2g	19%
Total Sugars	30.5g	
Protein	4.7g	

Tips: Cantaloupe and honeydew melon are both healthy options, but cantaloupe has more antioxidants.

LUNCH

Acorn Squash Soup

Prep time: 10 min	Cook time: 10 min	Servings: 2

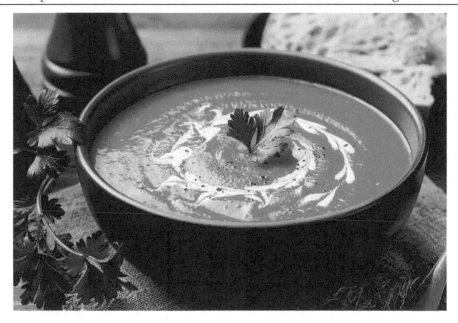

Ingredients

- 2 cups cooked acorn squash puree
- 1 cup cooked carrot puree
- 1 cup water
- 1 tsp ginger powder
- 1 strip of orange peel
- 1 tbsp chopped chives
- ¾ cup soy milk
- 1 tsp salt
- ¼ tsp ground black pepper

70

Directions

- Combine acorn squash, carrot, water, ginger powder, orange peel, and chives in a big pot.
- Bring to a boil, then reduce to a low heat and continue to cook for 10 minutes, stirring regularly to mix the flavors.
- Remove the orange peel from the dish. Remove the pan from the heat and stir in the soy milk.
- Season with salt and pepper to taste, and heat through without allowing the soup to boil.
- If preferred, drizzle a little more soy milk over each serving bowl and top with a sprinkling of lime zest.

NUTRITION FACTS (PER SERVING)

Calories	146	
Total Fat	1.8g	2%
Saturated Fat	0.2g	1%
Cholesterol	0mg	0%
Sodium	1257mg	55%
Total Carbohydrate	30.6g	11%
Dietary Fiber	5.1g	18%
Total Sugars	7g	
Protein	4.8g	

Tips: Acorn squash is high in soluble fiber that is easily tolerated by those with Crohn's disease.

Ginger Turkey Breasts

Prep time: 10 min	Cook time: 10 min	Servings: 2

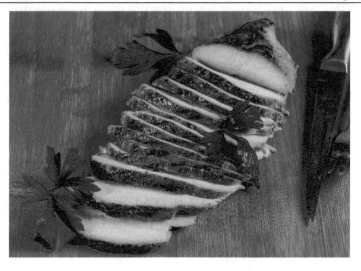

Ingredients

- *1 onion, sliced into thin wedges*
- *1 tbsp coconut oil*
- *1 tsp ginger powder*
- *2 boneless skinless turkey breasts*
- *1 tsp ground paprika*
- *salt & pepper to taste*

Directions

- Heat a pan over medium heat, add the oil. Add the onions and stir for 2-3 minutes, until brown.

- Remove the onions to a platter and add the turkey breast to the. Bake until golden brown on the outside. Cook covered for a few minutes, then flip to cook the other side.
- Sprinkle each side of the turkey with paprika, garlic powder, salt, and pepper, and continue to flip every couple of minutes, covering with a lid in between. This technique keeps the turkey breasts moist because the heat and liquid are trapped under the lid. Make a small slit in the turkey breast to see if it's thoroughly done – no longer pink in the center. If desired, top with additional paprika.
- Cut the turkey into bite-sized pieces. Serve with browned onions on top and mashed potatoes, if desired.

NUTRITION FACTS (PER SERVING)

Calories	188	
Total Fat	7.6g	10%
Saturated Fat	5.9g	30%
Cholesterol	0mg	0%
Sodium	3mg	0%
Total Carbohydrate	6.4g	2%
Dietary Fiber	1.7g	6%
Total Sugars	2.5g	
Protein	24.9g	

Tips: During a CD flare-up, high-fat foods might exacerbate or prolong your symptoms. Protein and other nutrients found in animal products, on the other hand, can avoid malnutrition. Lean meats such as skinless chicken and turkey are suitable examples.

Pan-Fried Flounder

Prep time: 10 min	Cook time: 25 min	Servings: 2

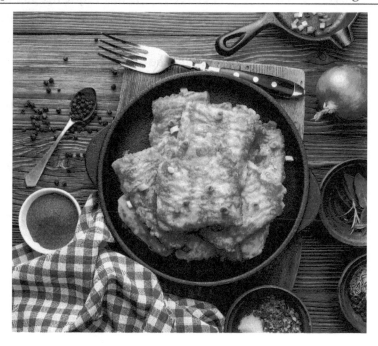

Ingredients

- 1 cup almond flour
- ½ tsp garlic, minced
- ¼ cup onions, chopped
- 1 tsp paprika
- ½ tsp ground caraway
- 4 (6-oz.) flounder filets
- sea salt and freshly ground black pepper
- 2 tbsp olive oil, divided

- *2 tbsp basil leaves, for garnish*
- *lemon wedges, for serving*

Directions

- Combine flour, garlic, onions, paprika, and caraway in a large mixing bowl.
- Season the flounder fillets with salt and pepper, then dip them in the flour mixture and shake off the excess. Place on a dish or a baking sheet.
- Heat the oil in a large nonstick skillet over medium heat. Cook for 3 to 4 minutes per side, until the crust is brown and the fish readily flakes with a fork. Continue with the remaining fillets.
- Serve immediately with lemon wedges and basil.

NUTRITION FACTS (PER SERVING)

Calories	407	
Total Fat	12.3g	16%
Saturated Fat	3.4g	17%
Cholesterol	100mg	33%
Sodium	707mg	31%
Total Carbohydrate	27.1g	10%
Dietary Fiber	1.7g	6%
Total Sugars	0.8g	
Protein	47.7g	

Tips: Omega-3 fatty acids are believed to be anti-inflammatory and easy on the stomach. This superfood also contains potassium, which aids fluid equilibrium in the body even when you have a flare. Other healthy and readily digestible seafoods are shrimps and white flaky fish like tilapia and flounder.

Stuffed Eggplants with Pork

Prep time: 10 min	Cook time: 35 min	Servings: 2

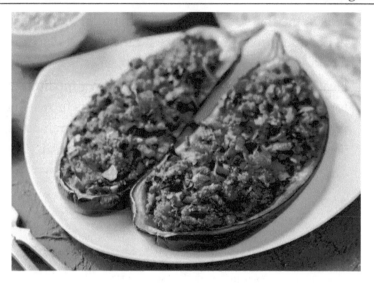

Ingredients

- 2 large eggplants, halved lengthwise
- 1 tsp olive oil
- 1 cup ground turkey
- ¼ cup panko bread crumbs
- ¼ cup shredded goat cheese
- ½ cup shredded gouda cheese
- 1 tsp garlic, powder
- ¼ cup chopped fresh cilantro

Directions

- Preheat the oven to 350 ° F.

- Slice eggplants lengthwise and scoop out the insides into a large mixing bowl.
- Heat the oil in a large skillet over medium heat. Add ground meat and cook for 6 minutes, or until seared.
- Add breadcrumbs, ½ cup goat cheese, gouda, garlic, and cilantro to a large mixing bowl.
- Fill the eggplants halves with the mixture and top with the remaining ¼ cup goat cheese.
- Bake for 15 minutes, or until eggplants are well cooked and cheese has browned.

NUTRITION FACTS (PER SERVING)

Calories	240	
Total Fat	10.9g	14%
Saturated Fat	4.5g	23%
Cholesterol	35mg	12%
Sodium	285mg	12%
Total Carbohydrate	21.5g	8%
Dietary Fiber	4.2g	15%
Total Sugars	6.7g	
Protein	16.9g	

Tips: A lot of individuals with Crohn's disease have digestive problems, so avoid foods that are high in fat, such as rib-eye steaks, pulled pork, beef brisket and fatty burgers. You should also avoid foods like pork sausage, hot dogs, and bacon since they are high in fat.

Panko-Crusted Salmon

Prep time: 10 min	Cook time: 17 min	Servings: 2

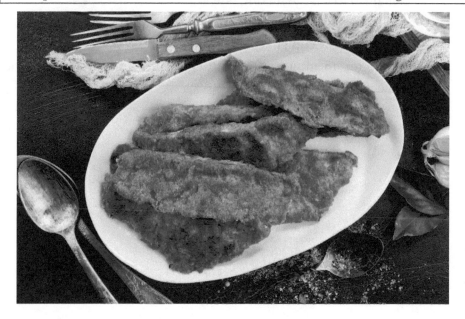

Ingredients

- 2 (5 ounce) salmon fillets
- ½ tsp salt, divided
- ¾ tsp freshly ground black pepper, divided
- ¼ cup coconut flour
- 1 large egg
- 1 cup unseasoned bread crumbs
- 1 tsp chopped chives
- ½ tsp basil
- ½ tsp garlic powder

Directions

- Using paper towels, pat the salmon fillets dry to remove any excess moisture. Season the fillets with a quarter tsp of salt and a quarter tsp of black pepper.
- Preheat your oven to 400 ° F. Prepare a sheet pan and lightly grease it with cooking spray or cover with baking paper.
- Add flour to 1 shallow bowl, whisk the egg in another shallow bowl, then add the bread crumbs to a third bowl. Add chives, basil, garlic powder, and the remaining salt and black pepper to the bread crumbs and stir to combine.
- Coat each fish fillet in flour one at a time, then eggs and finally bread crumbs. As you continue to coat all of the fillets, lay them on the prepared sheet pan.
- Put in the oven and bake for 16 to 18 minutes, or until the fillets are cooked through, opaque, and easily flake with a fork.

NUTRITION FACTS (PER SERVING)

Calories	435	
Total Fat	25.8g	33%
Saturated Fat	4.2g	21%
Cholesterol	75mg	25%
Sodium	172mg	7%
Total Carbohydrate	23.6g	9%
Dietary Fiber	2.3g	8%
Total Sugars	0.2g	
Protein	27.4g	

Tips: Salmon, tuna, and herring all include a lot of healthy omega-3 fatty acids, which may aid with Crohn's disease symptoms. Omega-3 fatty acids have anti-inflammatory effects and may help alleviate the aggravation that causes your symptoms to intensify.

Roasted Catfish with Basil

Prep time: 10 min	Cook time: 25 min	Servings: 2

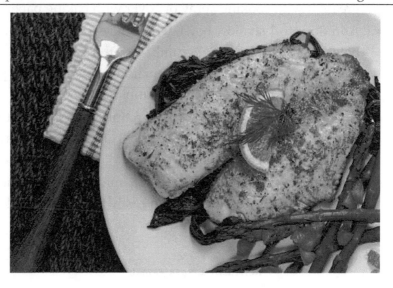

Ingredients

- 2 catfish filets (about 6oz. each)
- 1 tsp chipotle pepper powder
- ½ tsp dried basil
- ½ tsp garlic minced
- ¾ tsp caraway
- ¼ tsp chili powder
- 1 tbsp olive oil

Directions

- Preheat the grill to medium and lightly oil the grill grate.

- If you do not have a grill, use a pan and heat it over medium heat.
- Dry the fish with a paper towel.
- Mix all the seasonings and coat the fish generously.
- Put on the grill or in a pan and grill for 3 minutes per side, or until the catfish flakes easily with a fork.
- Serve with red pepper *pico de gallo* and cilantro as a garnish.

NUTRITION FACTS (PER SERVING)

Calories	275	
Total Fat	14.5g	19%
Saturated Fat	2.1g	10%
Cholesterol	78mg	26%
Sodium	229mg	10%
Total Carbohydrate	1.3g	0%
Dietary Fiber	0.2g	1%
Total Sugars	0.1g	
Protein	34.9g	

Tips: Catfish is high in omega-3 fatty acids, which are good for your heart and veins health and may help fight Crohn's disease.

Boiled Turkey

Prep time: 10 min	Cook time: 1h 20 min	Servings: 4

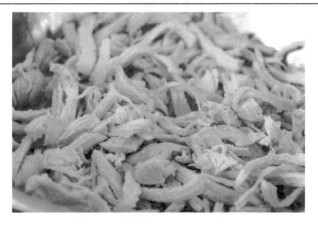

Ingredients

- *1 (3 pound) whole turkey*
- *1 large onion, halved - unpeeled*
- *3 parsnips, cut into chunks – unpeeled*
- *1 turnip cut into chunks*
- *2 stalks leek, cut into chunks*
- *1 tbsp allspice*
- *water to cover*

Directions

- Place the turkey with the onion, parsnips, leek and turnips in a large saucepan.
- Season with allspice and add water to cover.

- Cover the pot and bring to a boil, then reduce the heat and simmer for about 90 minutes or until the turkey comes off the bone.
- Remove the turkey and let it cool. Discard the bones and skin and chop or mince the meat. Serve immediately with cooked potatoes or your favorite vegetable as a side.

NUTRITION FACTS (PER SERVING)

Calories	341	
Total Fat	12.6g	16%
Saturated Fat	3.5g	17%
Cholesterol	151mg	50%
Sodium	166mg	7%
Total Carbohydrate	4.3g	2%
Dietary Fiber	1g	4%
Total Sugars	2g	
Protein	49.6g	

Tips: You may consider this meal bland and plain, but it will help you a lot if your symptoms worsen. It is easy to digest, as the meat is well cooked and will help you consume many important nutrients.

Herb Roasted Turkey

| Prep time: 10 min | Cook time: 30 min | Servings: 4 |

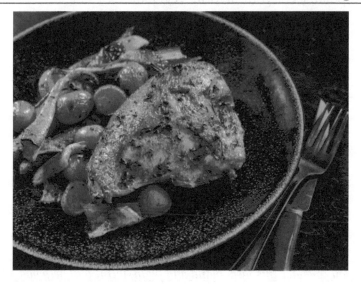

Ingredients

- 1 medium shallot
- 1 tsp garlic powder
- 1 tsp ground black pepper
- 2 tbsp garlic and herb seasoning blend
- ¼ cup butter
- 1-pound boneless, skinless turkey breasts

Directions

- Chop the shallot and garlic powder and put them in a bowl Add ground pepper, seasoning bland and butter and mix.

84

- Place the turkey breast in the marinade, cover and refrigerate for at least 4 hours or overnight.
- To cook, preheat the oven to 350 ° F.
- Cover a baking sheet with foil, place the marinated turkey breasts in the pan.
- Pour the rest of the marinade over the turkey and bake for 20 minutes. Grill for another 5 minutes to brown.

NUTRITION FACTS (PER SERVING)

Calories	337	
Total Fat	21.1g	27%
Saturated Fat	4.1g	21%
Cholesterol	101mg	34%
Sodium	99mg	4%
Total Carbohydrate	3.2g	1%
Dietary Fiber	0.8g	3%
Total Sugars	1.2g	
Protein	33.2g	

Tips: Turkey is comparable to chicken; however, turkey is slightly leaner than chicken. Breast meat, which is boneless and skinless, is the leanest part of the turkey you can eat.

Sweet Potato & Thyme Risotto

Prep time: 20 min	Cook time: 40 min	Servings: 6

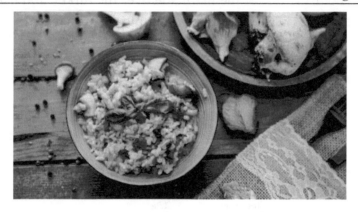

Ingredients

- 4 tbsp olive oil
- 2 sprig fresh thyme
- 1 large yellow onion, diced
- 2 cup pearled barley
- 2 large sweet potatoes, cut into a small dice
- 3 cups vegetable stock
- 3 cups water
- 1 tsp butter (optional)
- salt and black pepper, to taste

Directions

- In a 5-liter casserole dish, heat coconut oil over medium-high heat.

- When it starts to curl, add the thyme and cook for a minute, then add the onions. Cook, stirring constantly until the onions begin to turn transparent, about 2 minutes.
- Set the heat to medium, sprinkle the onions with a pinch of salt, stir and cover. Sweat for 8 minutes, stirring occasionally.
- Remove the lid, lower the heat to medium-high and add the barley. Mix and stir until the barley clicks against the side of the pan. Add the sweet potato and cook for another minute. Add the vegetable broth, water and bring to a boil. When the risotto has simmered, cover and lower the heat to low.
- Simmer for 20 minutes or until the barley is al dente and the sweet potatoes are tender. Stir in the butter vigorously. This will break the sweet potatoes a bit.
- Cover, turn off the heat and let the risotto stand for 5 minutes. Check the salt and consistency and serve.

NUTRITION FACTS (PER SERVING)

Calories	401	
Total Fat	12g	15%
Saturated Fat	9.3g	47%
Cholesterol	6mg	2%
Sodium	101mg	4%
Total Carbohydrate	67.4g	25%
Dietary Fiber	13.3g	48%
Total Sugars	6g	
Protein	8.8g	

Tips: Sweet potatoes are often touted as healthier than white potatoes, but in reality, both types can be very nutritious. While potatoes and sweet potatoes are comparable in calories, protein, and carbohydrates, white potatoes provide more potassium, while sweet potatoes are incredibly high in vitamin A.

Baked Halibut with Vegetables

| Prep time: 25 min | Cook time: 40 min | Servings: 2 |

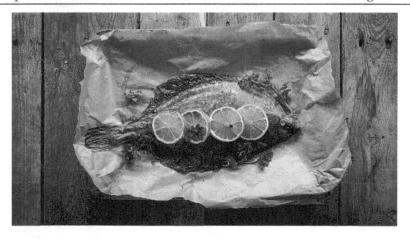

Ingredients

- 1 whole halibut scaled and cleaned
- 2 tbsp olive oil
- 1 tbsp lime juice
- 2 tsp sweet paprika
- 2 tbsp garlic powder
- ½ cup squash, cubed
- 2 tomatoes
- ½ eggplant, sliced
- 1 onion, quartered
- salt and pepper for seasoning

Directions

- Preheat oven to 400 ° F.

- Combine 1 tbsp olive oil, ½ tbsp lime juice, garlic powder, sweet paprika, salt and pepper in a mixing bowl. On each side of the fish, cut 3-4 diagonal cuts about 12 inches deep.
- Pour the remaining oil over the fish, sprinkle with salt and season it on the inside with the spice mixture.
- Toss the vegetables with the rest of the spice mixture. Make a bed of vegetables (excluding the tomatoes) on a sheet tray lined with aluminum foil.
- Arrange the fish and tomatoes on top. Cover the dish with aluminum foil and place in a preheated oven for 20-25 min to roast. Remove the foil and bake for another 10-15 min, or until the fish is just cooked through.

NUTRITION FACTS (PER SERVING)

Calories	372	
Total Fat	11.8g	15%
Saturated Fat	3.1g	16%
Cholesterol	81mg	27%
Sodium	503mg	22%
Total Carbohydrate	32.3g	12%
Dietary Fiber	7.5g	27%
Total Sugars	14g	
Protein	34.1g	

Tips: If you want a strong flavor, halibut is the way to go. It also has a thick and substantial texture to match. Cod, on the other hand, has a mild flavor and a flaky texture, which makes it an excellent option for cooking because of its versatility. They are both high in nutrients, vitamins, and minerals, and their nutritional profiles are complementary to one another. They are available in a number of cuts, and they are also a favorite dish among seafood lovers.

Tuscan Butter Roasted Chicken

Prep time: 15 min	Cook time: 1 h 25 min	Servings: 4

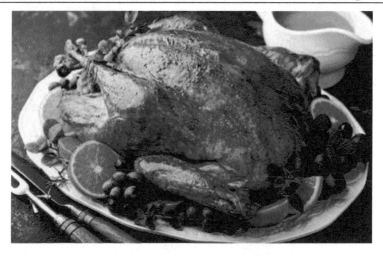

Ingredients

- *1 (3-lb.) whole chicken*
- *kosher salt and freshly ground black pepper*
- *1 lb. sweet potatoes, halved*
- *1 red onion, cut into wedges*
- *1 cup tomatoes, chopped*
- *½ zucchini, chopped*
- *a pinch of smoked paprika*
- *2 tbsp melted almond butter*
- *1 tsp garlic powder*
- *1 tsp dried basil*
- *¼ cup thinly sliced cilantro*

Directions

- Preheat the oven to 350°F and place a big skillet inside. Using paper towels, pat the turkey dry and season generously with salt and pepper.
- Toss sweet potatoes, zucchini, onion, and tomatoes in a large mixing bowl. Season with salt, pepper, and a pinch of smoked red pepper to taste.
- Combine the almond butter, garlic powder, and dried basil in a small bowl. Brush the chicken all over with the sauce.
- Carefully take the skillet from the oven and arrange the chicken in the center, followed by the vegetables. Bake for 1 hour and 15 minutes, or until the skin is crispy and golden and the internal temperature reaches 180°. During baking, pour over the chicken the pan juices several times, using a spoon.
- Serve cut into pieces over the vegetables, garnished with additional pan drippings and cilantro.

NUTRITION FACTS (PER SERVING)

Calories	922	
Total Fat	44.6g	57%
Saturated Fat	15.4g	77%
Cholesterol	334mg	111%
Sodium	445mg	19%
Total Carbohydrate	23.9g	9%
Dietary Fiber	5.6g	20%
Total Sugars	4.5g	
Protein	103.7g	

Tips: Poultry is high in brain-healthy amino acids and vitamins B6 and B12, which makes it an excellent source of lean protein for the diet. Choline and B vitamins have been linked to improved cognition and brain function.

Honey Flavored Shrimps

Prep time: 20 min	Cook time: 40 min	Servings: 4

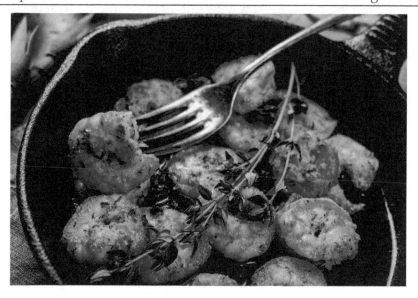

Ingredients

- *½ lb. shrimps, peeled and deveined*
- *kosher salt*
- *1 large egg, beaten*
- *½ cup potato starch*
- *olive oil for frying*
- *⅛ cup Greek yogurt*
- *2 tbsp maple syrup*
- *2 tbsp low-fat coconut cream*
- *thinly sliced leeks, for garnish*

Directions

- Using paper towels, pat the shrimps dry and season lightly with salt. In a shallow bowl, crack the egg and whisk. In another shallow bowl, add potato starch. Dip all shrimps in the egg bowl, then coat well with potato starch.
- Pour some olive oil into a large skillet and heat over medium heat. Fry the shrimps in batches, until golden brown, being careful to cover all sides, about 3 to 4 minutes.
- Place on a paper towel-lined plate after removing with a slotted spoon to drain extra fat.
- Whisk together Greek yogurt, maple syrup, and coconut cream in a medium mixing bowl.
- Serve the shrimps, garnished with leeks with a dipping sauce as a side.

NUTRITION FACTS (PER SERVING)		
Calories	617	
Total Fat	35.1g	45%
Saturated Fat	8.1g	40%
Cholesterol	332mg	111%
Sodium	402mg	17%
Total Carbohydrate	43.5g	16%
Dietary Fiber	3.6g	13%
Total Sugars	14.1g	
Protein	33.6g	

Tips: Shrimp cook quickly, so don't take your gaze away from them or they'll overcook and become chewy.

Turkey with Orange Roasted Zucchini

| Prep time: 20 min | Cook time: 25 min | Servings: 4 |

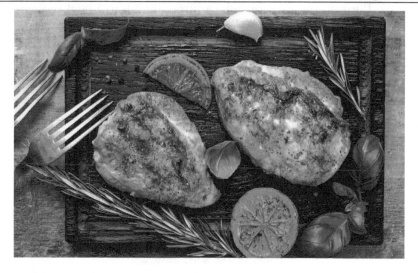

Ingredients

- ¾ lb. zucchini, cut into circles
- 1 tsp garlic powder
- 2 tbsp olive oil
- kosher salt and pepper
- 2 6-oz boneless, skinless turkey breast
- 1 tbsp lemon juice
- ½ lemon, cut into ½-inch pieces
- ½ cup water

Directions

- Preheat the oven to 425 ° F.

- Mix the zucchini and garlic with ½ tbsp of oil and ¼ tsp salt and pepper on a rimmed baking sheet and roast for 10 minutes.
- Lower the heat to 350 ° F. In a large skillet over medium-high heat, heat 1 tbsp of oil and cook turkey breast until golden brown, 3 to 5 minutes per side.
- Place the turkey on top of the zucchini, put in the oven and roast for 6 minutes, or until the turkey is cooked through and the zucchini is golden brown and soft.
- Heat the skillet over medium heat, add the remaining oil, followed by lemon pieces, lemon juice, and water and cook, stirring occasionally, for 2-3 minutes, or until beginning to color. Cook, stirring and scraping up any browned parts.
- Serve the turkey with zucchini as a side, covered with a few tbsp of sauce.

NUTRITION FACTS (PER SERVING)

Calories	384	
Total Fat	14g	18%
Saturated Fat	1.6g	8%
Cholesterol	64mg	21%
Sodium	110mg	5%
Total Carbohydrate	37.2g	14%
Dietary Fiber	5.7g	20%
Total Sugars	3.5g	
Protein	29.5g	

Tips: When roasting a whole turkey in the oven, the legs should be cooked longer than the breast. Remove the legs and return them to the oven after the breasts are done. This keeps the breasts moist – otherwise, you risk them being dry and chewy.

Carrot and Zucchini Soup

Prep time: 20 min	Cook time: 30 min	Servings: 4

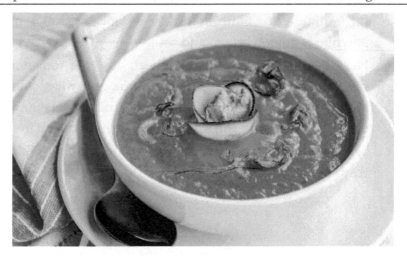

Ingredients

- 1 tsp coconut oil
- 1 small onion, finely chopped
- ½ lb. carrots, peeled and sliced
- ½ lb. zucchini, peeled and sliced
- ½ cup pumpkin, chopped
- ½ cup sweet potato, diced
- 1 tsp curry powder
- 2 cups low-sodium vegetable broth
- ⅛ cup fresh basil

Directions

- Sauté onions in a pot for 5 minutes or until just tender.

96

- Add the carrots and zucchini, sweet potato and pumpkin, then the curry powder.
- Stir for 1 to 2 minutes. Add the vegetable broth and bring to a boil.
- Reduce the heat and simmer for 20 minutes. In the end, add the chopped basil.
- Transfer the soup to a blender and mix gently, working in two batches.
- Serve and enjoy!

NUTRITION FACTS (PER SERVING)

Calories	100	
Total Fat	2.1g	3%
Saturated Fat	1.2g	6%
Cholesterol	0mg	0%
Sodium	438mg	19%
Total Carbohydrate	16.7g	6%
Dietary Fiber	3.6g	13%
Total Sugars	6.9g	
Protein	4.6g	

Tips: Steam expands quickly in a blender and can cause ingredients to splash all over or burn. To avoid this, fill the blender only a third of the way up, lift the lid and cover with a kitchen towel or aluminum foil while blending.

Broiled Tilapia with Ginger

Prep time: 4 h	Cook time: 10 min	Servings: 8

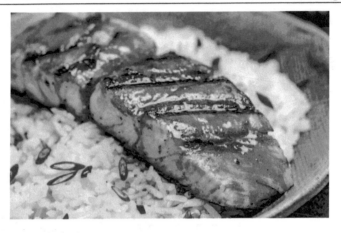

Ingredients

- 8 (6 ounces each) tilapia fillets
- 1 cup coconut aminos
- 1 tsp apple cider vinegar
- tbsp coconut oil
- tbsp fresh ginger, peeled and minced
- tsp garlic powder
- 1 cup leek finely chopped

Directions

- In a large glass bowl, combine the coconut aminos, vinegar, coconut oil, garlic powder, ginger and half the chopped leek.

- Place the tilapia in a large zippered bag, pour the marinade liquid into the bag, wring out any excess air, and seal it. Marinate the tilapia in the refrigerator for 2 to 4 hours.
- Preheat the grill for 5 minutes. Remove the fillets from the bag and place them skin side down on a baking sheet covered with a silicone baking mat. Place the pan on the top rack of your oven (or under the grill if you have a separate grill) and cook for 7-8 minutes, or until the fillets are flaky but still sag slightly when pressed.
- While the fillets are cooking, pour the remaining marinade into a saucepan and bring it to a boil. Then, simmer and reduce while the fillets are cooking.
- Serve the tilapia with the reduced marinade and garnish with the remaining leeks or herbs of your choice.

NUTRITION FACTS (PER SERVING)

Calories	250	
Total Fat	11.5g	15%
Saturated Fat	6.6g	33%
Cholesterol	55mg	18%
Sodium	79mg	3%
Total Carbohydrate	11g	4%
Dietary Fiber	0.9g	3%
Total Sugars	0.9g	
Protein	24.1g	

Tips: Avoid using glass cookware when cooking or if a recipe calls for adding liquid to a hot pot as the glass may explode. Even though this indicates that they are oven or heat resistant, tempered glass products can - and sometimes do.

Spiced Salmon and Shrimps with Thyme

| Prep time: 10 min | Cook time: 20 min | Servings: 4 |

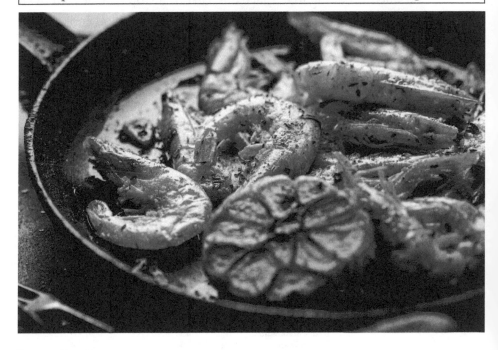

Ingredients

- 1 tbsp canola oil
- 2 tsp garlic powder (or 2 crushed garlic cloves)
- 3 large red bell peppers, chopped
- ½ tsp dried thyme
- ½ pound salmon
- ¼ pound large shrimp, peeled and deveined
- salt to taste

- *1 tbsp dried rosemary, or to taste*

Directions

- Heat the oil in a skillet over medium heat.
- Add the garlic, being careful not to burn the garlic. Add the red bell peppers and mix well. Add 1 tsp of thyme.
- Add the salmon and shrimps into the pan. Season with salt and dried rosemary to taste.
- Cover the pan and cook for 3 minutes. Flip the salmon and season with salt and additional rosemary (to taste). Cover again and cook for another 3 minutes.
- Remove the lid and cook until the juice has evaporated slightly, 2 to 3 minutes.

NUTRITION FACTS (PER SERVING)		
Calories	182	
Total Fat	5.7g	7%
Saturated Fat	0.9g	4%
Cholesterol	96mg	32%
Sodium	141mg	6%
Total Carbohydrate	7.7g	3%
Dietary Fiber	2g	7%
Total Sugars	4g	
Protein	25.9g	

Tips: Similar to salmon, shrimps also carry several health benefits. They are a great protein source, rich in omega 3 fatty acids. Shrimps are also a great source of vitamins, minerals and several important antioxidants our bodies need to function normally.

Garlic Chicken Meatballs

| Prep time: 10 min | Cook time: 15 min | Servings: 2 |

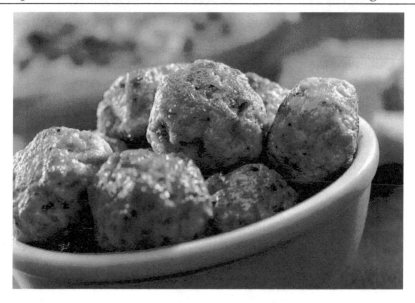

Ingredients

For the meatballs

- *½ lb. ground chicken*
- *¼ cup bread crumbs*
- *⅛ cup freshly grated goat cheese*
- *1 small onion, finely chopped*
- *1 large egg*
- *1 tsp garlic powder*
- *1 tbsp freshly chopped basil*
- *1 tbsp finely chopped leek*

- *1 tbsp soy milk*
- *kosher salt and freshly ground black pepper*
- *2 tbsp butter*
- *½ cup water and tomato sauce mixture*

Directions

- Preheat the oven to 350 ° F.
- Mix together ground chicken, bread crumbs, cheese, onion, egg, garlic powder, basil, leeks, milk, salt, and pepper in a large mixing basin. Make 112" balls out of the mixture.
- Melt the butter in a large skillet over medium heat. Sear the meatballs on all sides until golden brown, about 5 minutes. Cover the skillet with water and tomato sauce and cook until the meatballs are cooked through, about 6 minutes or so.
- Serve over baked spaghetti squash, garnished with basil and extra goat cheese.

NUTRITION FACTS (PER SERVING)

Calories	397	
Total Fat	24.2g	31%
Saturated Fat	7.1g	35%
Cholesterol	179mg	60%
Sodium	342mg	15%
Total Carbohydrate	13.6g	5%
Dietary Fiber	1.3g	5%
Total Sugars	2.3g	
Protein	35.8g	

Tips: An excellent meatball is made up of around half meat and half breadcrumbs. If desired, you can skip the sauce part of the recipe and eat the fried meatballs as are, dipping them in low-fat yogurt or sour cream.

Best-Ever Pork Meatloaf

| Prep time: 15 min | Cook time: 1 h 20 min | Servings: 2 |

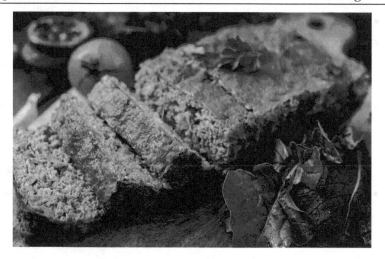

Ingredients

- *1 tbsp olive oil*
- *1 chopped onion*
- *1 tsp garlic powder*
- *1 tbsp finely chopped thyme*
- *1 tsp chopped basil leaves*
- *kosher salt and freshly ground black pepper*
- *2 lb. ground lean pork*
- *¾ cup panko bread crumbs*
- *½ cup soy milk*
- *1 egg*
- *⅓ cup tomato puree*

- *2 tbsp honey*

Directions

- Preheat the oven to 325°F. Spray a big deep baking dish with cooking spray or line with baking paper.
- Heat the oil in a large skillet over medium heat. Add the onion and cook, stirring occasionally, 2-3 minutes. Add the garlic powder and herbs, then cook for 1 minute or until aromatic. Remove from the heat and set aside to cool.
- Combine ground pork, panko breadcrumbs, milk, egg, and cooked onion with herbs in a large mixing bowl. Season with salt and pepper to taste.
- Form the meat mixture into a loaf in the prepared baking dish.
- Stir tomato puree and honey together in a small bowl, then brush over the loaf. Bake for 1 hour and 20 minutes, or until the internal temperature reaches 160°.

NUTRITION FACTS (PER SERVING)

Calories	435	
Total Fat	21.2g	27%
Saturated Fat	3.8g	19%
Cholesterol	187mg	62%
Sodium	515mg	22%
Total Carbohydrate	21.4g	8%
Dietary Fiber	1.5g	5%
Total Sugars	9.9g	
Protein	45.6g	

Tips: During cooking, cover a single big meatloaf with aluminum foil to keep it moist, but leave it exposed for the last 15 minutes of baking. Meatloaf freezes well, either raw for later cooking or cooked and frozen for reheating.

Ground Chicken Potato Skillet

| Prep time: 10 min | Cook time: 20 min | Servings: 2 |

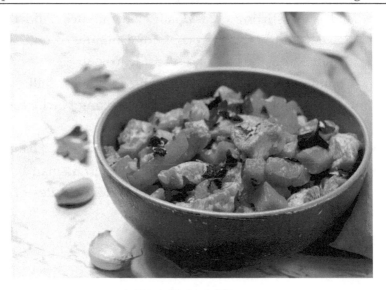

Ingredients

- 2 tbsp olive oil
- ½ pound lean ground chicken
- 1 tsp garlic powder (or 1 clove minced garlic)
- ½ cup onions, sliced
- ½ cup Anaheim peppers, diced
- ¾ cup potato, cooked and diced
- salt and freshly ground black pepper
- a pinch of paprika - optional
- ½ cup shredded goat cheese
- fresh cilantro, for garnishing (optional)

Directions

- Heat the olive oil in a cast-iron skillet over medium-high heat.
- Combine the ground chicken, onions and garlic in a mixing bowl. Put into a skillet and cook for about 5 minutes, stirring occasionally. Use a wooden spoon to split up the meat.
- Add the Anaheim peppers, potatoes and paprika and stir. Season with salt and pepper. Cook for 5 minutes, covered in the skillet. Don't forget to stir from time to time.
- Preheat the oven to 400 ° F. Add the shredded goat cheese over the cooked meat and veggies and bake for 5 minutes, until the cheese melts. Garnish with fresh cilantro.

NUTRITION FACTS (PER SERVING)

Calories	363	
Total Fat	9.4g	12%
Saturated Fat	1.4g	7%
Cholesterol	2mg	1%
Sodium	121mg	5%
Total Carbohydrate	60.1g	22%
Dietary Fiber	9.7g	35%
Total Sugars	18.5g	
Protein	12g	

Tips: Cooking chicken in the oven or stir-frying it with vegetables is the healthiest way to prepare it. Place the portions in a baking pan, drizzle with olive oil, and top with garlic, lemon, carrots, or whatever else you desire. Preheat the oven to 350°F and bake until golden brown.

Whole Roasted Flounder

Prep time: 20 min	Cook time: 40 min	Servings: 2

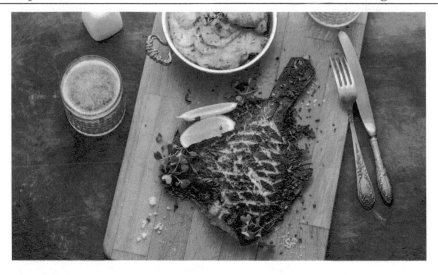

Ingredients

- 1 lime, cut in half and into 4 slices each half
- 1 (½ lb.) whole flounder, cleaned and butterflied
- 1 tbsp olive oil
- sea salt and freshly ground black pepper
- 6 sprigs fresh rosemary, divided, plus more for serving
- ½ onion, thinly sliced
- 4 tsp butter, sliced into pats

Directions

- Preheat the oven to 425 ° F and line a baking sheet with aluminum foil.

- With a paper towel, pat the outside and inside of the flounder, then coat the entire fish with oil and season with salt and pepper. Add 3 rosemary sprigs to the prepared baking sheet, then place lime slices and onion slices on top of the rosemary, evenly distributing the onion between the lime slices. Put the flounder on top, and cover with the butter and 3 additional rosemary sprigs.
- Fold up the top layer of foil to cover the fish and put it in the oven.
- Bake for 12 to 16 minutes, depending on the size of the fish, until flaky and tender. To test, carefully open the foil and use a fork to see if the fish flakes. Transfer the fish from the foil to a large plate. Remove the burnt lime and save the foil filled with cooking liquids.
- Serve with fresh lime juice, freshly chopped herbs, or cooked potatoes if desired.

NUTRITION FACTS (PER SERVING)

Calories	322	
Total Fat	20.3g	26%
Saturated Fat	7.3g	36%
Cholesterol	101mg	34%
Sodium	175mg	8%
Total Carbohydrate	5.1g	2%
Dietary Fiber	1.9g	7%
Total Sugars	0.8g	
Protein	30.4g	

Tips: Flounder fillets in a skillet: in a skillet over medium-high heat, warm the olive oil or butter. When a squirt of water sizzles on contact with the pan, it's ready. Place the fish in the heated pan, seasoned side down. Cook 2–3 minutes per side.

Garlic Feta Salmon

Prep time: 5 min	Cook time: 30 min	Servings: 2

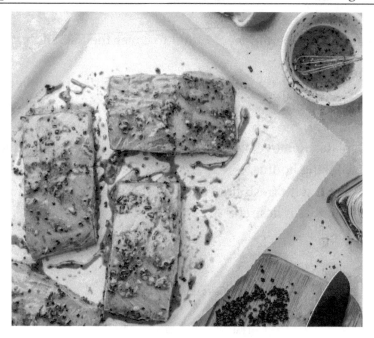

Ingredients

- ⅛ *cup olive oil*
- *2 salmon filets*
- *kosher salt and freshly ground black pepper*
- ¼ *cup freshly grated feta cheese*
- ⅛ *cup bread crumbs*
- *1 tsp garlic powder*
- *juice and zest of ½ orange*

Directions

- Preheat the oven to 400 ° F. On a large baking sheet, drizzle 2 tbsp oil. Season the salmon with salt and pepper.
- Combine the feta, bread crumbs, garlic, and orange zest on a big dish. Lay the fish in the mixture and press on all sides so that the mixture adheres well to the fish.
- Lay the fillets on a baking sheet.
- Drizzle the remaining oil and orange juice over the fish, put in the oven and bake for 15-20 minutes, or until golden brown and the fish flakes readily with a fork.

NUTRITION FACTS (PER SERVING)

Calories	255	
Total Fat	15.3g	20%
Saturated Fat	2.4g	12%
Cholesterol	58mg	19%
Sodium	221mg	10%
Total Carbohydrate	7.4g	3%
Dietary Fiber	0.8g	3%
Total Sugars	0.8g	
Protein	21.4g	

Tips: When you roast salmon fillets in the oven, you get a gorgeous, succulent fish that doesn't need to be watched all the time.

Creamed Kale Stuffed Tilapia

Prep time: 10 min	Cook time: 25 min	Servings: 2

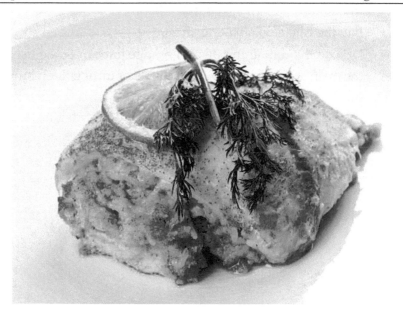

Ingredients

- *2 (6-oz.) tilapia fillets*
- *kosher salt and freshly ground black pepper*
- *¼ (8-oz.) block tofu, crumbled*
- *¼ cup shredded feta cheese*
- *¼ cup frozen kale, defrosted*
- *⅛ tsp garlic minced*
- *a pinch of sweet paprika*
- *1 tbsp ghee (or coconut) butter*

Directions

- Season the tilapia with salt and pepper. Combine tofu, feta, kale, garlic, and paprika in a large mixing bowl.
- Make a pocket in each fish fillet by cutting a slit with a paring knife. Stuff the mixture into the pockets evenly.
- Melt the butter in a large skillet over medium heat. Cook the fish fillets for 6 minutes, skin side down, until the fish is seared, then flip to the other side. Cook for another 6 minutes, or until the skin is crispy.

NUTRITION FACTS (PER SERVING)

Calories	362	
Total Fat	25.1g	32%
Saturated Fat	7.4g	37%
Cholesterol	96mg	32%
Sodium	193mg	8%
Total Carbohydrate	1g	0%
Dietary Fiber	0.2g	1%
Total Sugars	0.6g	
Protein	34.6g	

Tips: Cooking techniques that preserve the most nutrients and reduce the production of harmful chemicals while minimizing the loss of beneficial omega-3 fatty acids are generally considered to be the healthiest. Some of the technics we suggest include sous vide, microwaving, baking, steaming, and poaching your fish.

DINNER

Lime Ginger Meatballs

Prep time: 15 min	Cook time: 25 min	Servings: 2

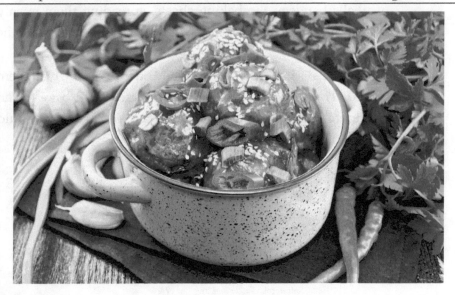

Ingredients

- *1-pound lean ground pork*
- *18 oz orange zest*
- *4 oz lime juice*
- *1 tbsp maple syrup*
- *2 tsp garlic powder*
- *2 tsp fresh ginger*
- *2 tsp sweet paprika*
- *2 tsp dried basil*
- *1 tsp kosher salt*
- *½ tsp black pepper*

Directions

- Preheat the oven to 400 ° F.
- Spray two dark-coated nonstick pans with cooking spray.
- Make the meatballs: combine all the ingredients in a bowl and mix well. Make 112" balls out of the mixture. Divide the meatballs between the baking sheets, spreading them evenly apart. Bake for 10 minutes in the upper and lower thirds of the oven.
- If the meatballs have already browned on the bottom, turn them around. Transfer the pans to opposing racks and bake for an additional 8 to 12 minutes, or until cooked through (should register 165 ° F in the center of meatballs).
- Serve garnished with fresh herbs and vegetables.

NUTRITION FACTS (PER SERVING)

Calories	237	
Total Fat	4.2g	5%
Saturated Fat	1.5g	7%
Cholesterol	22mg	7%
Sodium	351mg	15%
Total Carbohydrate	45.9g	17%
Dietary Fiber	0.7g	3%
Total Sugars	40.8g	
Protein	7g	

Tips: If preferred, add the meatballs to your favorite tomato or meat sauce and simmer the baked meatballs on low heat for about 10 minutes to achieve an extra moist and tender structure.

Creamy Tuscan Tempeh

Prep time: 15 min	Cook time: 15 min	Servings: 4

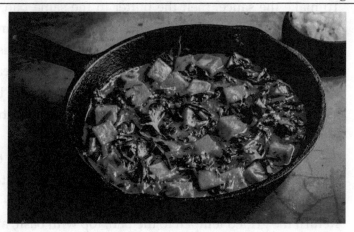

Ingredients

- *2 oz tempeh*
- *1 tsp olive oil*
- *1 tbsp ghee butter*
- *2 minced garlic cloves*
- *1 small onion, diced*
- *⅓ cup water*
- *5 oz. tomato puree*
- *2 cups low-fat coconut cream*
- *salt and pepper, to taste*
- *2 cups baby kale leaves*
- *¼ cup grated goat cheese*
- *1 tbsp fresh basil, chopped*

Directions

- In a large skillet, heat the oil over medium-high heat. Season the tempeh pieces on both sides with salt and pepper, then sear for 5 minutes on each side in a pan, flesh-side down first. Remove from the pan and set aside.
- To make the sauce, melt the butter in the same pan. Add the onion and garlic and fry until it is aromatic (1-2 min). Add tomato puree and fry for another minute to release flavor. Finally, add the water and let the sauce slightly decrease.
- Reduce the heat to low, add the coconut cream, and bring to a soft simmer, stirring from time to time. Season with salt and pepper.
- Stir in the kale and goat cheese, allowing it to wilt in the sauce. Allow the cream sauce to simmer for another minute or until the cheese has completely melted.
- Return the grilled tempeh to the pan, top with basil, and gently stir. Serve over steamed vegetables or rice.

NUTRITION FACTS (PER SERVING)		
Calories	118	
Total Fat	7.3g	9%
Saturated Fat	3.1g	16%
Cholesterol	30mg	10%
Sodium	416mg	18%
Total Carbohydrate	5.3g	2%
Dietary Fiber	0.5g	2%
Total Sugars	3.9g	
Protein	8.1g	

Tips: Refrigerate leftovers for up to 5 days in an airtight container. It's delicious cold, but you can reheat it by covering it with a splash of water or chicken stock and cooking it on the stove.

Cajun Herbed Aroma Tuna

Prep time: 10 min	Cook time: 20 min	Servings: 2

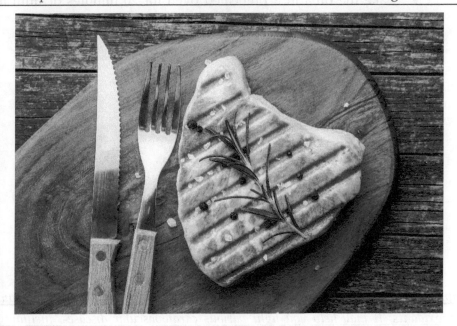

Ingredients

- 1 pound tuna
- 5 dried marjoram leaves
- 1 tbsp dried rosemary
- 1 pinch ground Cajun spice
- 1 pinch ground chili
- 1 rosemary string

Directions

- Preheat the oven to 350 ° F.

- Cut a piece of foil, large enough to fold all the tuna. Spray one side of the foil with cooking spray.
- Place the tuna on the prepared side of the foil. Sprinkle with the seasonings and add the rosemary string. Fold the foil over the tuna to enclose it.
- Bake the tuna in a preheated oven for 20 minutes or until it flakes easily with a fork.

NUTRITION FACTS (PER SERVING)

Calories	310	
Total Fat	14.4g	18%
Saturated Fat	2.2g	11%
Cholesterol 1	00mg	33%
Sodium	101mg	4%
Total Carbohydrate	2g	1%
Dietary Fiber	1.3g	5%
Total Sugars	0.1g	
Protein	44.4g	

Tips: Tuna is a low-cost protein source, abundant in omega 3 fatty acids and antioxidants. It may help you fight various cardiovascular diseases, including heart disease.

Mexican Tofu and Squash

Prep time: 10 min	Cook time: 25 min	Servings: 4

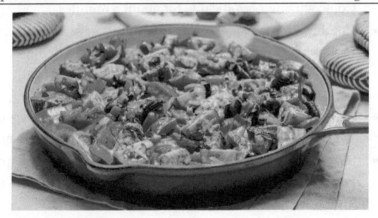

Ingredients

- 1 tbsp olive oil
- 1 small onion, finely chopped
- 1 small jalapeno, chopped
- 1 tsp garlic, minced
- 1 lb. tofu, cut into 1" pieces
- 1 tbsp cumin, divided
- 1 tsp salt and ground black pepper
- 1 eggplant, diced
- 7 oz. tomatoes, chopped
- 1 tsp taco seasoning
- ⅓ cup shredded Parmesan cheese
- ½ cup leek, chopped
- ½ cup basil, chopped

Directions

- Preheat a large (12-inch) deep skillet over low-medium heat, swirling the oil to coat it. Sauté the onion, garlic jalapeno for 3 minutes, stirring occasionally. Add the tofu to the side of the skillet and season with ½ tsp cumin, 1 tsp salt and black pepper. Cook, stirring periodically, for about 5 minutes.
- Combine tomatoes, eggplant pieces, taco seasoning, and the remaining cumin in a large mixing bowl. Add to the skillet and cook for 10 minutes over low-medium heat, stirring occasionally.
- Add the cheese and cover and heat for a few minutes, or until the cheese has melted. Put the chopped leek and basil on top.
- Serve immediately, either alone or with brown rice or quinoa. Sour cream, cilantro, and black olives can be added as a garnish after the cheese has been added.

NUTRITION FACTS (PER SERVING)

Calories	136	
Total Fat	3.6g	5%
Saturated Fat	0.4g	2%
Cholesterol	44mg	15%
Sodium	451mg	20%
Total Carbohydrate	7.7g	3%
Dietary Fiber	2.3g	8%
Total Sugars	3.6g	
Protein	19.5g	

Tips: Those who are lactose intolerant will benefit from hard cheeses like Cheddar and Parmesan since they contain less lactose, a milk sugar that may cause discomfort and bloating. In addition, goat cheese contains almost no lactose. Even if you can't eat any other dairy products, you may be able to tolerate one of the mentioned cheeses while on Crohn's disease diet.

Teriyaki Tempeh and Zucchini

Prep time: 10 min   Cook time: 20 min   Servings: 4

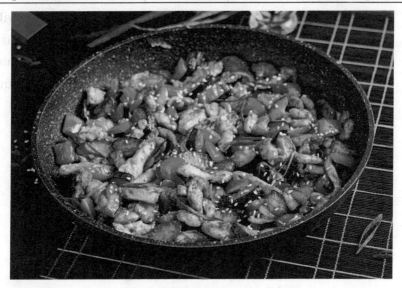

Ingredients

- 2 tbsp of olive oil
- 1 ½ lbs. zucchini, chopped into small florets
- 2 tempeh cut into 1" cubes
- 2 tsp garlic powder
- 1 tbsp ginger powder
- 1 tbsp finely chopped chives

Teriyaki Sauce

- 2 tbsp coconut aminos
- 3 tbsp barley malt syrup

- *2 tbsp apple cider vinegar*
- *1 tbsp rice flour*

Directions

- For the sauce, combine all the ingredients in a mixing bowl. Set aside after everything is well incorporated.
- Preheat a deep skillet over medium-high heat and coat with oil.
- Add the zucchini, tempeh, garlic, ginger, and chives and cook for 8 minutes, stirring frequently, to allow a bit of browning.
- Whisk together the teriyaki sauce and the water, then pour over the tempeh and heat for 2 minutes, or until thickened.

NUTRITION FACTS (PER SERVING)

Calories	297	
Total Fat	9g	11%
Saturated Fat	0.9g	5%
Cholesterol	88mg	29%
Sodium	588mg	26%
Total Carbohydrate	16.2g	6%
Dietary Fiber	3.4g	12%
Total Sugars	8.9g	
Protein	38.6g	

Tips: Refrigerate in an airtight container for up to 3-4 days.

Korean Ground Pork and Barley Bowls

Prep time: 10 min	Cook time: 20 min	Servings: 4

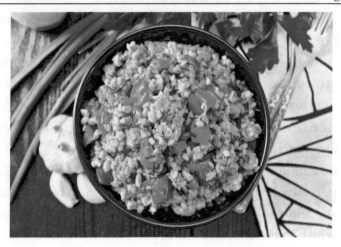

Ingredients

- 2 cups cooked barley
- 1 tbsp oil
- 1 lb. ground lean pork
- 1 large onion diced
- 1 tsp ginger powder
- 2 garlic cloves, minced
- ½ jalapeno, diced
- 1 zucchini, diced
- 1 tomato, diced (optional)
- 4-5 tbsp coconut aminos
- 1 tbsp apple cider vinegar
- 3 tbsp date paste

- *ground black pepper to taste*
- *a pinch of sweet paprika*
- *2 tbsp of freshly chopped leeks*

Directions

- Heat the oil over medium heat in a wok and add the pork. Cook for about 5-7 minutes, breaking up the ground pork and stirring regularly. If desired, drain the fat.
- Add the onion, ginger, jalapeno and garlic at the end of browning ground pork. Cook, stirring periodically, for 2-3 minutes.
- Add zucchini pieces, mushrooms and tomatoes and cook for another 5 minutes.
- Combine the coconut aminos, apple cider vinegar, Date Paste, pepper, and paprika in a mixing bowl. Add to the meat mixture, stir and cook for 1 minute. Remove the pan from the heat and whisk in the chopped leeks.
- To serve, fluff the barley with a fork and top it with Korean ground pork.

NUTRITION FACTS (PER SERVING)

Calories	244	
Total Fat	8.4g	11%
Saturated Fat	2.3g	11%
Cholesterol	68mg	23%
Sodium	785mg	34%
Total Carbohydrate	15.6g	6%
Dietary Fiber	2.4g	8%
Total Sugars	10.1g	
Protein	25.3g	

Tips: Refrigerate leftovers for up to 5 days in an airtight container. I recommend storing the meat and vegetable mixture separately from the rice so that the grain does not absorb all of the delectable juices.

Garlicky Chicken

Prep time: 10 min	Cook time: 20 min	Servings: 4

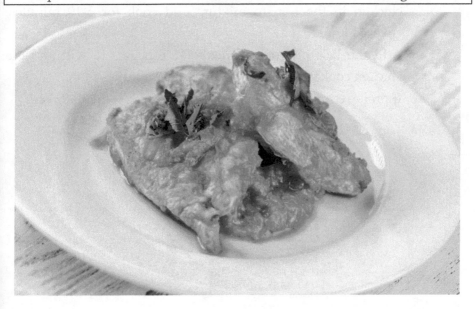

Ingredients

- *1 tbsp olive oil*
- *1 garlic clove, minced*
- *2 strips orange zest*
- *1 8-oz can tomato puree*
- *2-pound chicken breasts*
- *1 cup kale*
- *⅛ cup crumbled goat cheese (or Parmesan cheese)*

Directions

- In a large skillet over medium heat, heat the oil.
- Whisk in the garlic and orange zest until they begin to brown, about 1 minute.
- Add the tomato puree and bring it to a low simmer. Place the chicken in the tomato mixture and cook for 5-10 minutes, covered.
- Add the kale and stir, until the kale begins to wilt and the chicken cooked throughout, about 5-10 minutes more.
- If preferred, top with cheese and serve with some flatbread.

NUTRITION FACTS (PER SERVING)

Calories	203	
Total Fat	7.5g	10%
Saturated Fat	2.5g	12%
Cholesterol	232mg	77%
Sodium	673mg	29%
Total Carbohydrate	6.6g	2%
Dietary Fiber	1.2g	4%
Total Sugars	2.9g	
Protein	26.9g	

Tips: Cook the chicken to the right temperature, as undercooking will result in toughness, while overcooking will result in moisture loss, making the chicken drier. Allow 10 to 15 minutes for the roasted chicken to rest before carving it, to allow the fluids to flow evenly throughout the meat.

Katsu Tofu Cutlet

Prep time: 10 min	Cook time: 20 min	Servings: 4

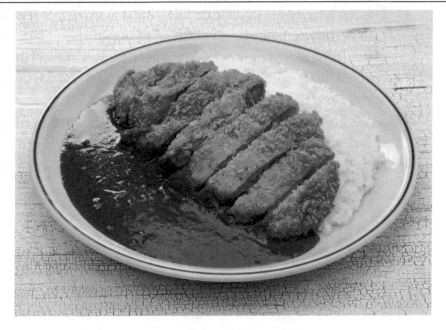

Ingredients

- 1 large egg
- 1 cup rice flour
- 2 tbsp olive oil
- kosher salt and pepper
- 1 lb. tofu, cut into pieces
- 2 tbsp apple cider vinegar
- 1 tbsp fresh lemon juice
- 1 tsp ginger powder

- *1 tsp maple syrup*

Directions

- Preheat the oven to 400 ° F. In a small bowl, whisk the egg. Combine rice flour, oil and salt and pepper in a second bowl or plate.
- Dip the tofu pieces in the egg, allowing any excess to drip off, then in the rice flour, gently pushing to help it stick. Place on a rack, arranged in a rimmed baking sheet. Repeat until all tofu is covered, then roast for 20 to 25 minutes, or until golden brown and cooked through.
- Meanwhile, combine the vinegar, lemon juice, ginger, maple syrup, and ½ tsp of salt and pepper in a mixing bowl.
- Drizzle the sauce over the tofu pieces and serve with white rice.

NUTRITION FACTS (PER SERVING)

Calories	497	
Total Fat	16.4g	21%
Saturated Fat	3.8g	19%
Cholesterol	176mg	59%
Sodium	499mg	22%
Total Carbohydrate	44.5g	16%
Dietary Fiber	3.2g	11%
Total Sugars	5.9g	
Protein	40.5g	

Tips: Sandwich the tofu between many layers of paper towel-lined plates and weigh it from the top to avoid the soggy tofu syndrome. Leave for 10 minutes and drain extra liquid.

Orange and Basil Turkey

Prep time: 10 min	Cook time: 20 min	Servings: 4

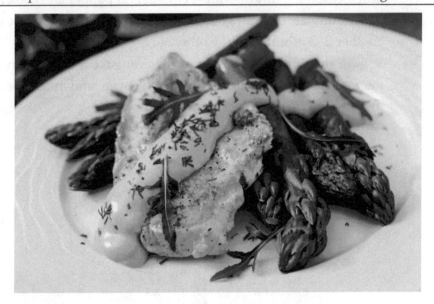

Ingredients

- 1 lb. asparagus, trimmed as much as possible
- 2 tbsp freshly cut and roughly chopped basil, divided
- 2 tbsp coconut oil, divided
- kosher salt and black pepper
- ½ c. grated feta, divided
- 1 ½ lb. turkey breasts
- 1 orange, halved

Directions

- Preheat the oven to 425 ° F.

- Toss asparagus and half of the basil with 1 tbsp of oil and ¼ tsp of salt and pepper on a rimmed baking sheet, then top with ¼ cup feta cheese. Put in the oven and roast on the bottom rack in the oven for 10 minutes, or until golden brown and tender.
- In a large oven-safe skillet, heat the remaining oil over medium heat. Season the turkey with ¼ tsp salt and pepper and cook for 3 to 4 minutes, or until golden brown on the bottom. Cook for another 2 -3 minutes on the other side.
- Toss in the remaining basil and the orange, cut side down, to the skillet. Transfer the skillet to the oven and roast for 10 minutes or until the meat is cooked through.
- Serve on a plate garnished with the remaining cheese.

NUTRITION FACTS (PER SERVING)

Calories	697	
Total Fat	49.7g	64%
Saturated Fat	21.9g	110%
Cholesterol	146mg	49%
Sodium	149mg	6%
Total Carbohydrate	20g	7%
Dietary Fiber	7.7g	28%
Total Sugars	8.8g	
Protein	45.1g	

Tips: Some people have trouble digesting asparagus due to its tough skin. However, if you pill the skin off or use only the tips of this wonderful vegetable, you might benefit from its many vitamins, minerals and antioxidants. Make sure to cook it well.

Roasted Potatoes with Garlic and Parsley and Rosemary

Prep time: 10 min	Cook time: 25 min	Servings: 4

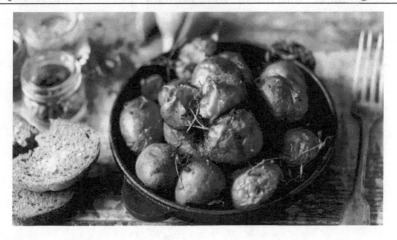

Ingredients

- ¾ pound small potatoes, peeled
- 4 garlic cloves
- 2 tsp coconut oil
- 2 tsp chopped fresh rosemary
- ⅛ tsp salt
- ¼ tsp ground black pepper
- 2 tsp butter
- 2 tbsp chopped fresh parsley

Directions

- Preheat oven to 400 F.
- Lay a large baking dish with parchment paper.

- To a large bowl, add the whole potatoes, garlic cloves, coconut oil, rosemary, salt and pepper. Mix until the potatoes are coated with oil and spices.
- Place the potatoes on the prepared baking dish, then cover and bake for 20-25 minutes.
- Remove the lid or foil. Flip the potatoes and cook them, uncovered, until the potatoes are tender and lightly browned (about 25 minutes).
- Put in a bowl and mix with butter. Sprinkle with parsley and serve.

NUTRITION FACTS (PER SERVING)

Calories	103	
Total Fat	4.4g	6%
Saturated Fat	3.2g	16%
Cholesterol	5mg	2%
Sodium	94mg	4%
Total Carbohydrate	15.1g	5%
Dietary Fiber	1.9g	7%
Total Sugars	0.9g	
Protein	1.9g	

Tips: Potatoes can be a lifesaver if you are suffering from Crohn's disease. Just avoid potato skins, which are rich in fiber and may cause stomach issues. So make sure to peel it off and cook or bake potatoes well.

Roasted Root Vegetable Soup

| Prep time: 15 min | Cook time: 1 h | Servings: 4 |

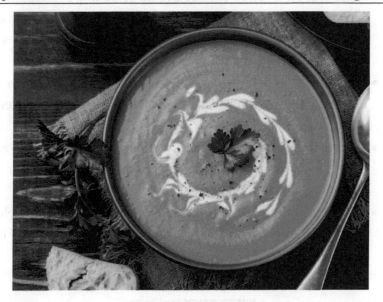

Ingredients

- ½ tbsp olive oil
- ½ small pumpkin peeled, seeded, chopped
- 1 beet, peeled and chopped
- 1 sweet potato, peeled and chopped
- 1 small turnip, peeled and chopped
- 2 shallots, chopped
- 2 bay leaves
- 2 marjoram sprigs
- 2 sage sprigs

135

- *1 cup water*
- *2 cup vegetable stock*
- *salt and black pepper*

Directions

- Preheat the oven to 400 ° F. In a large mixing bowl, combine the chopped veggies with the olive oil. Spread them out in a single layer on a big baking tray. Combine the herbs and sprinkle them over the veggies.
- Unless the vegetables are soft earlier, roast for about 50 minutes. During the cooking process, you should turn the vegetables a few times.
- Transfer the vegetables to a large pot, discard the herbs and add the stock and water. Bring to a boil, then decrease the heat to low and let it simmer for 10 minutes.
- Using a food processor or blender, puree the vegetables until smooth. Add salt and pepper to taste and extra water, if desired.

NUTRITION FACTS (PER SERVING)		
Calories	204	
Total Fat	13g	17%
Saturated Fat	1.8g	9%
Cholesterol	0mg	0%
Sodium	82mg	4%
Total Carbohydrate	21.8g	8%
Dietary Fiber	6.4g	23%
Total Sugars	5.5g	
Protein	2.1g	

Tips: If a soup tastes bland in the bowl, try adding acid instead of salt. A touch of lemon or lime, as well as a dollop of yogurt or sour cream, helps brighten the dish.

Five Spice Turkey

Prep time: 5 min	Cook time: 20 min	Servings: 2

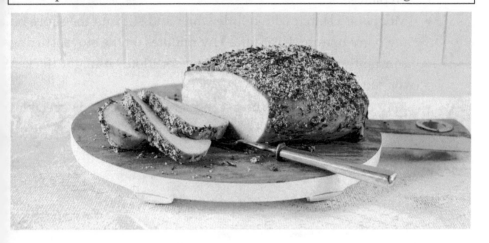

Ingredients

- *2 turkey breasts*
- *2 tbsp coconut aminos*
- *2 tbsp maple syrup*
- *½ tsp garlic powder*
- *½ tsp smoked paprika*
- *½ tsp onion powder*
- *½ tsp allspice*
- *1 tbsp potato starch*

Directions

- Preheat the oven to 380 ° F.

- In an oven-safe dish, combine the maple syrup, coconut aminos, and allspice, garlic, paprika and onion powder, then add the turkey breast and coat them in the sauce. Cook for 20 minutes in the oven.
- Remove the turkey breast from the oven and arrange the steaks on plates.
- Mix potato starch with a little water and stir into the sauce on the pan's bottom. Heat for a few minutes on the stove, stirring constantly. If necessary, add some cornflour, it might thicken the sauce slightly.
- Pour the sauce over the breast and serve with cooked vegetables or potatoes.

NUTRITION FACTS (PER SERVING)

Calories	282	
Total Fat	8.2g	10%
Saturated Fat	3g	15%
Cholesterol	75mg	25%
Sodium	1092mg	47%
Total Carbohydrate	22.7g	8%
Dietary Fiber	3.7g	13%
Total Sugars	17.6g	
Protein	25.9g	

Tips: Allspice is a spice produced from the dried berries of the myrtle-family member Pimenta dioica that produces allspice. It tastes like a mix of cinnamon, nutmeg and cloves. It's hard to imagine Thanksgiving without allspice because of the way it tastes.

Barley with Acorn Squash and Spinach

Prep time: 5 min	Cook time: 20 min	Servings: 2

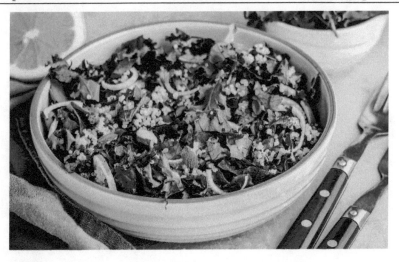

Ingredients

- 1 ¼ cups acorn squash, roasted or cooked
- ½ cup barley
- 1-½ cups cooked spinach, shredded
- 1 tbsp avocado oil
- 1 tsp garlic powder
- salt and ground black pepper to taste

Directions

- Cut the squash into ¼-inch cubes.
- Cook barley according to package directions in salted boiling water. Drain once done, but save some of the water.

- Meanwhile, in a big pan, sauté the spinach and garlic in the avocado oil, along with 1-2 tbsp of leftover water from the barley cooking. Cook for 1-2 minutes, or until the spinach reaches your desired softness.
- In a bowl, combine together barley, acorn squash and spinach and serve.

NUTRITION FACTS (PER SERVING)

Calories	279	
Total Fat	7.9g	10%
Saturated Fat	1g	5%
Cholesterol	0mg	0%
Sodium	31mg	1%
Total Carbohydrate	47g	17%
Dietary Fiber	6.4g	23%
Total Sugars	4.8g	
Protein	7.2g	

Tips: How to cook barley? Pearl barley does not need to be soaked before cooking and becomes soft as it cooks. Pot barley tastes the best after being soaked in cold water overnight and then cooked in three parts liquids to one part grains.

Trout Stir Fry

Prep time: 10 min	Cook time: 20 min	Servings: 4

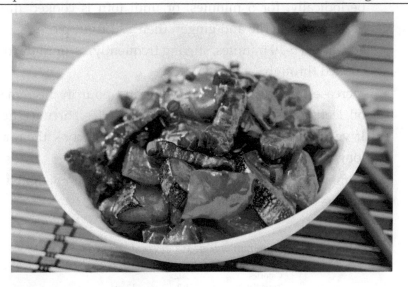

Ingredients

- *1.5 lbs. trout fillet cut into 1" cubes*
- *3 tbsp coconut aminos*
- *11 oz zucchini, sliced into small cubes*
- *handful of mushrooms, sliced*
- *2 cups tofu, sliced*
- *1 tbsp garlic powder*
- *1 tbsp ginger powder*
- *2 tsp coconut oil, divided*
- *1 tsp soy sauce*
- *¼ cup leeks, chopped*

Directions

- Combine trout pieces and 2 tbsp of coconut aminos in a medium mixing dish and set aside to marinate for 10 min.
- Heat 1 tsp of coconut oil over medium heat in a medium-sized pan. Add tofu, zucchini and mushrooms and cook, stirring periodically, for 5 minutes, or until tofu is cooked through. Season with garlic and ginger, then add trout pieces. Cook for additional 5-10 minutes, stirring frequently, or until the trout is cooked through.
- Increase the heat to medium-high and pour in the remaining oil, leeks and soy sauce. Cook for 2-3 minutes, stirring regularly. If you prefer your vegetables to be softer, cook them a little longer.
- Remove from heat, mix gently, and serve immediately with quinoa or your favorite stir-fry noodles.

NUTRITION FACTS (PER SERVING)

Calories	202	
Total Fat	9.2g	12%
Saturated Fat	1.3g	7%
Cholesterol	50mg	17%
Sodium	507mg	22%
Total Carbohydrate	7.1g	3%
Dietary Fiber	2.5g	9%
Total Sugars	1.8g	
Protein	24.7g	

Tips: Zucchini can be replaced with asparagus tips, peas, or broccolini. Also, no need to thaw frozen stir fry vegetables from a bag – go for fresh ones instead.

Easy Lime Baked Tempeh

Prep time: 15 min	Cook time: 20 min	Servings: 4

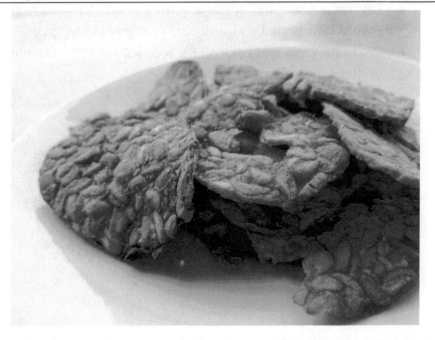

Ingredients

- 16 ounces tempeh
- 2 tbsp olive oil
- juice of ½ lime
- sea salt
- black pepper
- ½ tsp onion powder
- 1 tsp fresh oregano leave
- ½ cup freshly grated Parmesan

Directions

- Preheat the oven to 425 ° F.
- Pour the oil and lime juice into a small rectangle baking dish.
- Slice the tempeh thinly and season it with salt, pepper, oregano, and onion powder on both sides.
- Lay on a plate and sprinkle with cheese. Any stray cheese should be collected and sprinkled on top of the tempeh.
- Put in the oven and bake on the top rack for 10-12 minutes, or until the tempeh has browned.

NUTRITION FACTS (PER SERVING)

Calories	163	
Total Fat	7.8g	10%
Saturated Fat	1.5g	8%
Cholesterol	53mg	18%
Sodium	317mg	14%
Total Carbohydrate	0.6g	0%
Dietary Fiber	0.1g	0%
Total Sugars	0.1g	
Protein	23.2g	

Tips: To remove the bitterness from the tempeh, place it in a rimmed skillet or saucepan with 1 inch of water. Tempeh steams for 10-12 minutes, flipping midway. Rinse, dry, and slice into thin pieces.

Creamy Eggplant Soup

Prep time: 15 min	Cook time: 20 min	Servings: 2

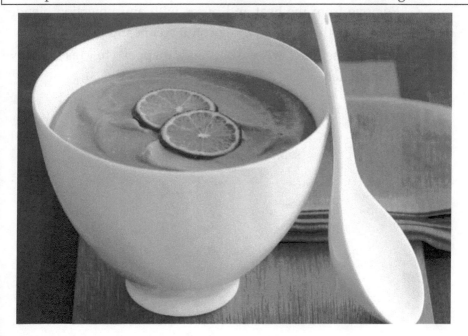

Ingredients

- 8 oz low-fat chicken broth
- 8 oz water
- ¼ small onion, quartered
- 2 cloves garlic
- 1-½ medium eggplant, cut into chunks
- 1 tbsp low-fat coconut cream
- kosher salt and black pepper to taste

Directions

- In a large pot over medium heat, bring the chicken broth, onion, garlic, and eggplant to a boil.
- Reduce the heat to low, cover, and cook for about 20 minutes, or until the vegetables are soft.
- Remove from the heat and puree with an immersion blender until smooth, then add the coconut cream and puree again.
- Finally, season with salt and pepper to taste. Serve immediately.

NUTRITION FACTS (PER SERVING)

Calories	42	
Total Fat	1.3g	2%
Saturated Fat	0.6g	3%
Cholesterol	3mg	1%
Sodium	209mg	9%
Total Carbohydrate	6.7g	2%
Dietary Fiber	1.8g	7%
Total Sugars	3.1g	
Protein	2.4g	

Tips: Always add raw vegetables to the pot to allow the taste to permeate the soup. Bring everything to a boil, then reduce to low heat. It's done when all ingredients are soft, which can take anywhere from 20 minutes to 3 hours, depending on the ingredients.

Barbecue Baked Carrots

Prep time: 15 min	Cook time: 30 min	Servings: 4

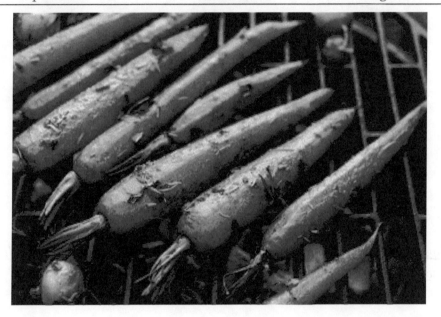

Ingredients

- *8 medium carrots*
- *4 tsp coconut oil*
- *4 tbsp sour cream*
- *1 leek, sliced*

Directions

- Rub each carrot with a little oil and salt, then wrap in a double layer of aluminum foil.

- As soon as the charcoal turns red, place the carrots directly on it. Cook for 15 minutes, flip with tongs, then cook for another 15 minutes. Take one out, unwrap it, and see if it's done.
- Peel off the top of the foil from each carrot, open it and cover it with a tbsp of sour cream and a few slices of leek.

NUTRITION FACTS (PER SERVING)

Calories	273	
Total Fat	4.6g	6%
Saturated Fat	1.9g	10%
Cholesterol	5mg	2%
Sodium	47mg	2%
Total Carbohydrate	46g	17%
Dietary Fiber	6.2g	22%
Total Sugars	4.8g	
Protein	12.4g	

Tips: Carrots include many vitamins and antioxidants that help fight Crohn's disease. Cooked and baked carrots are easier to digest than raw ones.

Roasted Vegetables

Prep time: 10 min	Cook time: 30 min	Servings: 4

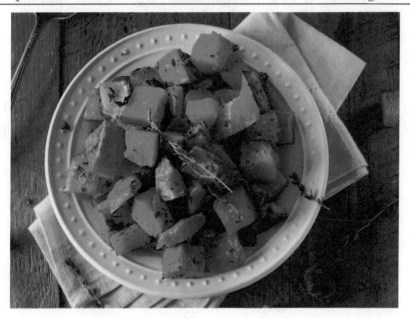

Ingredients

- *2 cups sweet potatoes, cut into 1-inch dice*
- *1 medium green bell pepper, chopped into bite-size pieces*
- *1 cup zucchini, split in half and sliced*
- *½ cup eggplant, split in half and sliced*
- *½ cup carrots, sliced*
- *1 cup green beans, cut into small pieces*
- *½ cup beet, diced*
- *1 tbsp garlic powder*
- *¼ cup olive oil*

- *2 tsp dried basil*
- *½ tsp black pepper*
- *1 tsp apple cider vinegar*

Directions

- Add water to a saucepan and bring to a boil. Add the sweet potatoes and cook for 15 min, until tender.
- Combine the cooked potatoes with bell peppers, zucchini, eggplant, carrot, beet, green beans, garlic powder, canola oil, and basil. Mix thoroughly.
- Spread the vegetables on a broiler pan, season with black pepper, and broil for 12 to 15 min, or until the edges are slightly browned. During the cooking process, stir a few times.
- Toss the veggies with the apple cider vinegar in a large mixing dish. Serve at room temperature or heated.

NUTRITION FACTS (PER SERVING)

Calories	178	
Total Fat	12.9g	17%
Saturated Fat	1.9g	9%
Cholesterol	0mg	0%
Sodium	8mg	0%
Total Carbohydrate	15.4g	6%
Dietary Fiber	2.2g	8%
Total Sugars	2.1g	
Protein	2.5g	

Tip: To preserve the juices in your broiler pan and make cleanup easier, line it with aluminum foil.

Slow Cooker Pork

Prep time: 15 min	Cook time: 6 h	Servings: 6

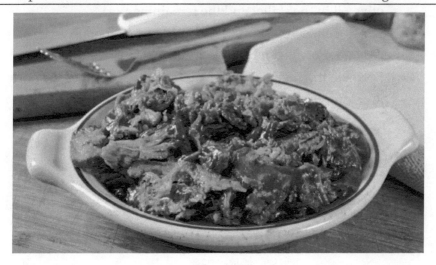

Ingredients

- kosher or sea salt to taste
- ¼ tsp black pepper divided
- pork chops
- 1 tbsp olive oil, divided
- ½ cup water
- 1-½ tbsp tomato paste
- ⅛ cup potatoes starch (optional)
- ¼ tsp ground coriander
- ¾ cup pitted capers

Directions

- Combine ¼ tsp pepper and ¼salt and season the meat.
- In a large skillet over medium-high heat, heat ½ tbsp oil; add half of the pork. Cook for 3 minutes on each side, or until golden brown. Place in a slow cooker. Rep with the remaining ½ tbsp olive oil in the skillet and the remaining pork.
- Stir together the water, tomato puree, potato starch, and coriander using a whisk. Pour the mixture over the pork.
- Sprinkle the capers and more pepper on the top of the pork.
- Cook for 6 hours on low heat, covered.

NUTRITION FACTS (PER SERVING)

Calories	165	
Total Fat	7g	9%
Saturated Fat	1.4g	7%
Cholesterol	95mg	32%
Sodium	189mg	8%
Total Carbohydrate	2.8g	1%
Dietary Fiber	0.1g	0%
Total Sugars	0.1g	
Protein	22.5g	

Tips: One of the most typical slow cooker blunders is adding liquid to every recipe when you really don't need it unless you're creating a soup or stew. As a result, any liquid from your ingredients (vegetables, meat, poultry) will leak into the crockpot.

2-WEEK DIET PLANS

1st Week Meal Plan

Day	Breakfast	Snack	Lunch	Dinner
1	Potato & Spinach Frittata	Beet Hash	Acorn Squash Soup	Cajun Herbed Aroma Tuna
2	Sweet Potato Omelette	Banana Protein Smoothie	Ginger Turkey Bread	Creamy Tuscan Tempeh
3	Easy Oatmeal Pancakes	Beet & Kiwi Smoothie	Herb Roasted Turkey	Mexican Tofu and Squash
4	Breakfast Muffins	Tofu & Egg Muffins	Tuscan Butter Roasted Chicken	Tofu Stir Fry
5	Easy Quiche	Melon Smoothie	Honey Flavored Shrimps	Slow Cooker Pork
6	Acorn Squash Breakfast Bowl	Honeydew Smoothie	Carrot and Zucchini Soup	Five Spice Turkey
7	Carrot Muffins	Scrambled Eggs	Creamed Kale Stuffed Tilapia	Barley with Acorn Squash and Spinach

2nd Week Meal Plan

Day	Breakfast	Snack	Lunch	Dinner
1	Carrot Muffins	Melon Smoothie	Garlic Feta Salmon	Katsu Tofu Cutlet
2	Tempeh Pancakes	Honeydew Smoothie	Ground Chicken Potato Skilled	Teriyaki Tempeh and Zucchini
3	Easy Quiche	Avocado and Oatmeal Smoothie	Broiled Tilapia with Ginger	Orange and Basil Turkey
4	Breakfast Muffins	Potato & Spinach Frittata	Boiled Turkey	Creamy Eggplant Soup
5	Easy Oatmeal Pancakes	Beet Hash	Sweet Potato & Thyme Risotto	Roasted Vegetables
6	Sweet Potato Omelette	Banana Protein Smoothie	Baked Halibut with Vegetables	Korean Ground Pork and Barley Bowls
7	Pork, Sweet Potato & Egg Bake	Beet & Kiwi Smoothie	Roasted Catfish with Basil	Barbecue Baked Carrots

Made in United States
Troutdale, OR
11/01/2023

14213139R00086